4.00

Health and Fitness

A Guide to a Healthy Lifestyle

D1566982

Laura E. Bounds, M.S.

Dottiedee Agnor, M.S.

Gayden S. Darnell, M.S.

Emma S. Gibbons, Ph.D.

Texas A&M University

KENDALL/HUNT PUBLISHING COMPANY
4050 Westmark Drive   Dubuque, Iowa 52002

Copyright © 2000 by Kendall/Hunt Publishing Company

ISBN 0-7872-6858-5

Printed in the United States of America
10 9 8 7 6 5 4 3 2 1

"To laugh often and much; to win the respect of intelligent people and the affection of children; to earn the appreciation of honest critics and endure the betrayal of false friends; to appreciate beauty, to find the best in others; to leave the world a little better, whether by a healthy child, a garden patch or a redeemed social condition; to know even one life has breathed easier because you have lived. This is the meaning of success."

—Ralph Waldo Emerson

Contents

Acknowledgments

The authors would like to acknowledge the following individuals for their invaluable contributions in the writing of *Health and Fitness: A Guide to a Healthy Lifestyle*:

Julie Barber, M.S.

Roger Bounds, M.S.

Kirstin Brekken Shea, M.S.

William Coady, M.S.

Tamara Franks, M.A.G.

Melinda Grant, M.S.

Janet Hardcastle, M.S.

Sandra Kimbrough, M.S.

Ernie Kirkham, M.S.

Susan Lowy, M.S.

Dianne Maddox, M.S.

Martha Muckleroy, M.Ed.

Linda Mullen, M.D.

Jeremy Nelms, M.S.

Christine Reeves, M.S.

Teresa Wenzel, M.S.

Brian Wigley, M.S.

Nicole Wilkerson, M.S.

We also acknowledge with appreciation the continuing guidance and support from the expert review panel:

Robert Armstrong, Ph.D.

Danny Ballard, Ed.D

Susan Bloomfield, Ph.D.

Maurice Dennis, Ph.D.

Jerry Elledge, Ph.D.

Margaret Griffith, M.S.

Linda Mullen, M.D.

B.E. Pruitt, Ed.D.

Jack Wilmore, Ph.D.

Special thanks to:
Roger Bounds, Richard Darnell, Kathy Durkin, Alicia Jordan, and Kristin Slagel for their guidance, support, and input.

Without the technical knowledge of Walter Suarez, the development of the Powerpoint presentation and the contribution it makes to the text would not have been possible.

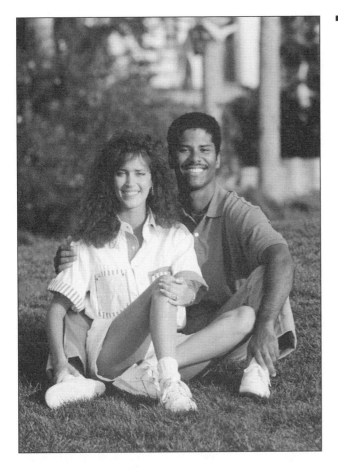

Chapter One

Defining Health

"Take care of your body with steadfast fidelity. The soul must see through these eyes alone, and if they are dim, the whole world is clouded."

—Johann Wolfgang Von Goethe

OBJECTIVES

Students will be able to:

- define health

- define wellness

- list and describe the five components of wellness

- establish a link between preventative behaviors and wellness

- introduce and explain the significance of *Healthy People 2000: National Health Promotion and Disease Prevention*

- list *Healthy People 2000* objectives for Priority Areas contained within the *Health & Fitness* text

Health is a universal trait. The World Health Organization defines *health* as "A state of complete physical, mental, and social well-being and not merely the absence of disease or infirmity." Webster's Dictionary offers "the condition of being sound in body, mind, or spirit; especially: freedom from physical disease or pain…the general condition of the body" as a definition of health. However, health also has an individual quality. Health is very personal and it is unique to each individual.

Early on, definitions of health revolved around issues of sanitation and personal hygiene. Today the definition of health has evolved from a basis of mere physical health or absence of disease, to a term that encompasses the emotional, mental, social, spiritual, and physical dimensions of an individual.

This current, positive approach to health is referred to as wellness. *Wellness* is a process of making informed choices that will lead one, over a period of time, to a healthy lifestyle that should result in a sense of well-being.

Components of Wellness

Wellness emphasizes each individual's potential and responsibility for his or her own health. It is a process in which a person is constantly moving either away from or toward their most favorable level of health. Wellness results in the adoption of low-risk, health enhancing behaviors. The adoption of a wellness lifestyle requires a focus on choices that will enhance the individual's potential to lead a productive, meaningful, and satisfying life. Assessment of one's behaviors in the following dimensions is essential to living a balanced life:

- *Emotional.* An individual who is emotionally healthy is able to enjoy life despite unexpected challenges and problems. Effectively coping with life's difficulties is essential to good health. Negative emotions can affect the immune system and result in chronic stress (see Chapter 3) which in turn can lead to serious illness and potential death.

- *Mental.* The mind is a very powerful tool. It has substantial influence over the body. To be healthy, it is important to be able to recognize which thoughts result in smiles and positive feelings and which thoughts cause frowns or muscle tightness and tension.

- *Social.* Social health is an individual's ability to relate to and interact with others. Socially healthy people are able to communicate and interact with other people—they are respectful and caring of their family, friends, neighbors, and associates.

- *Spiritual.* Spiritual health helps a person achieve a sense of inner peace, satisfaction, and confidence. It gives the sense that all is right with the world. A person's ethics, values, beliefs, and morals can contribute to his or her spiritual health.

- *Physical.* Physical health is comprised of cardiovascular fitness, muscular strength and endurance, flexibility (Chapter 2), and body composition (Chapter 8). It is the component most often associated with a person's health.

Through wellness, an individual manages the range of their lifestyle choices. How a person chooses to behave with regard to spirituality, fitness (Chapter 2), sexuality (Chapter 5), alcohol use (Chapter 7),

Figure 1.1
The Components of Wellness

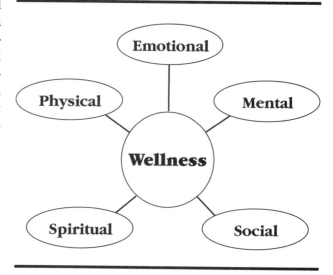

drug use (Chapter 7), and nutrition (Chapter 8) will determine, to a great degree, how 'well' that individual will live.

Wellness and Stress

Stress is the nonspecific response to demands which are placed on the body. 'Nonspecific response' alludes to the production of the same physiological reaction regardless of the type of stress placed on the body. Stress reactions are unique to each individual. The same event might be perceived as highly stressful and draining to one person but simply stimulating and exciting to another person.

Stress reactions are a person's physical and emotional responses to stimuli. These responses can be positive or they can be negative. *Eustress* is a positive stress that produces a state of well-being.

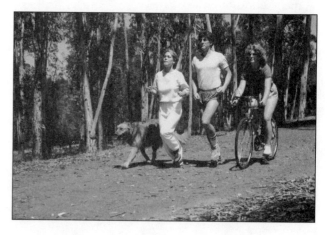

It is a healthy component of daily life. Examples of activities that might initiate a positive stress response include competitive sports, dating, the birth of a baby, or a long awaited vacation. Eustress can help channel nervous energy into a top notch performance.

Distress is negative stress. It is a physically and mentally damaging response to the demands placed upon the body. Distress is associated with changes that interrupt the natural flow of life. Schoolwork, loss of a job, or moving away from family are examples of activities that may produce a negative stress response in some individuals.

Stress has historically been seen as a support for the idea of 'survival of the fittest.' When an individual looks primarily at the reactions of the body to stressors, the realization occurs that many of the adaptations and defense mechanisms which are innate to humans are specific responses to stress. With this in mind, the necessity of stress (such as thriving on less sleep during final exams or being socially active in a new environment) becomes obvious.

Healthy People 2000

There are four major factors that influence personal health. The four factors are heredity, environment, access to professional health care personnel, and personal behavior.

Personal behaviors that result in prevention of disease or premature death are the primary focus of this text. Prevention is a key factor in promoting wellness. Its importance is made clear in *Healthy People 2000: National Health Promotion and Disease Prevention.* Healthy People 2000 was first developed in 1979 and is reformulated each decade to review the progress of the health of Americans during the last part of the century. According to the Department of Health and Human Services, "Healthy People 2000 defines the nation's health agenda for the current decade through more than 300 objectives in disease prevention and health promotion."

Each of the chapters in *Health and Fitness: A Guide to a Healthy Lifestyle* corresponds to a Priority Area within *Healthy People 2000.* Some Priority Areas within *Healthy People 2000* are beyond the scope of this text. However, Priority Areas contained in the text and a list of the objectives for those Priority Areas are as follows:

Priority Area: *Physical Activity and Fitness*— Text Chapter 2

Year 2000 Objectives

- Reduce coronary heart disease deaths
- Reduce overweight prevalence
- Preserve independent functioning in older adults
- Increase moderate physical activity
- Increase vigorous physical activity
- Reduce sedentary lifestyle
- Increase activities that enhance muscular strength, endurance, and flexibility
- Increase sound weight loss practices
- Increase participation in school physical education
- Increase activity level in school physical education
- Increase worksite fitness programs
- Increase availability and accessibility of community fitness facilities
- Increase physical activity counseling by primary care providers

Priority Area: *Heart Disease and Stroke*— Text Chapter 3

Year 2000 Objectives

- Reduce coronary heart disease deaths
- Reduce stroke deaths
- Reduce end-stage renal disease
- Increase control of high blood pressure
- Increase therapeutic actions by those with high blood pressure
- Reduce mean serum cholesterol
- Reduce prevalence of high blood cholesterol
- Increase therapeutic actions by those with high blood cholesterol
- Reduce dietary fat intake
- Reduce prevalence of overweight
- Increase moderate physical activity
- Reduce prevalence of cigarette smoking
- Increase blood pressure screening
- Increase blood cholesterol screening
- Increase initiation of appropriate diet and/or drug therapy for high blood cholesterol

- Increase worksites offering blood pressure and cholesterol education
- Increase the proportion of clinical laboratories meeting the accuracy standard for cholesterol measurement

Priority Area: *Violent and Abusive Behavior*—Text Chapter 4

Year 2000 Objectives

- Reduce homicides
- Reduce suicides
- Reduce weapon-related deaths
- Reverse rising incidence of child abuse
- Reduce physical abuse of women by male partners
- Reduce assault injuries
- Reduce rape and attempted rape
- Reduce adolescent suicide attempts
- Reduce physical fighting among youth
- Reduce weapon-carrying by youth
- Reduce inappropriate storage of weapons
- Improve emergency room protocols to identify, treat, and refer suicide attempters, survivors of sexual assault and spouse, elder, and child abuse
- Improve child death review systems
- Improve evaluation and follow-up of abused children
- Improve emergency housing for battered women and their children
- Improve school programs for conflict resolutions skills
- Increase violence prevention programs
- Increase suicide prevention in jails
- Enact in 50 States laws for proper firearm storage

Priority Area: *Unintentional Injuries*—Text Chapter 4

Year 2000 Objectives

- Reduce unintentional injury deaths
- Reduce unintentional injuries
- Reduce motor vehicle crash deaths
- Reduce fall-related deaths
- Reduce drowning deaths

- Reduce residential fire deaths
- Reduce hip fractures among older adults
- Reduce poisonings
- Reduce head injuries
- Reduce spinal cord injuries
- Reduce disabilities associated with head and spinal cord injuries
- Increase use of occupant protection systems
- Increase use of helmets
- Increase safety belt and helmet use laws
- Enact laws on handgun design
- Increase installation of fire sprinklers
- Increase functional smoke detectors
- Provide injury prevention instruction in schools
- Increase use of protective headgear at sporting events
- Improve roadway safety design standards
- Increase counseling on injury prevention
- Extend emergency medical services and trauma systems
- Limit motor vehicle crash deaths to 5.5 per 100,000
- Extend to 50 States bicycle helmet laws
- Enact in 50 States laws for proper firearm storage
- Increase number of States with a graduated drivers licensing system to 35

Priority Area: *Family Planning*—Text Chapter 5

Year 2000 Objectives

- Reduce pregnancies among adolescents
- Reduce unintended pregnancies
- Reduce the prevalence of infertility
- Encourage postponement of sexual activity among adolescents
- Increase abstention from sexual activity among sexually active adolescents
- Increase the use of contraception that both effectively prevents pregnancy and provides barrier protection against disease among sexually active young people
- Increase the effectiveness with which family planning methods are used

- Improve discussion of human sexuality
- Increase counseling about pregnancy options
- Increase availability of appropriate preconception care and counseling
- Increase appropriate counseling and referral services for HIV infection and STDs
- Increase contraceptive use among females ages 15–44

Priority Area: *Sexually Transmitted Diseases*—Text Chapter 5

Year 2000 Objectives

- Reduce gonorrhea
- Reduce *Chlamydia trachomatis* infections
- Reduce primary and secondary syphilis
- Reduce congenital syphilis
- Reduce genital herpes and genital warts
- Reduce the incidence of pelvic inflammatory disease
- Reduce hepatitis B infection
- Reduce repeat gonorrhea infection
- Increase adolescent postponement of sexual intercourse
- Increase condom use
- Increase clinic services for HIV infection and STDs
- Increase education in schools about STDs
- Increase correct management of STD cases
- Increase counseling on prevention of HIV and STDs
- Increase partner notification of exposure to STDs
- Increase abstention from sexual activity among sexually active adolescents
- Increase HIV and other STD information, education, and counseling on college and university campuses

Priority Area: *HIV Infection*—Text Chapter 5

Year 2000 Objectives

- Confine incidence of diagnosed AIDS cases
- Confine prevalence of HIV infection
- Encourage adolescent postponement of sexual intercourse

- Increase condom usage
- Increase the proportion of drug abusers in treatment programs
- Increase the proportion of intravenous drug abusers using uncontaminated drug paraphernalia
- Reduce transfusion-transmitted HIV infection
- Increase testing for HIV infection
- Increase primary care and mental health care provider counseling on HIV and other sexually transmitted diseases
- Increase HIV education in schools
- Provide HIV education in colleges and universities
- Increase outreach to drug abusers
- Increase the proportion of clinics that screen, diagnose, treat, counsel, and provide partner notification services for HIV infection and bacterial STDs
- Reduce occupational exposure to bloodborne infections
- Increase abstention from sexual activity among sexually active adolescents
- Increase the proportion of business that implement HIV/AIDS education programs
- Increase linkages between primary care clinics and substance abuse treatment programs

Priority Area: *Cancer*—Text Chapter 6

Year 2000 Objectives

- Reverse the rise in cancer deaths
- Slow the rise in lung cancer deaths
- Reduce deaths from breast cancer
- Reduce uterine cervix cancer deaths
- Reduce colorectal cancer deaths
- Reduce cigarette smoking
- Reduce dietary fat intake
- Increase intake of fiber-containing foods
- Increase the proportion of people who limit sun exposure and use sunscreens
- Increase the proportion of primary care providers who routinely counsel patients about tobacco use cessation, diet modification, and cancer screening
- Increase the proportion of women age 50 and older who have received a clinical breast

exam and mammogram within the preceding 1 to 2 years

- Increase Pap tests
- Increase fecal occult blood testing and proctosigmoidoscopy
- Increase oral, skin, and digital rectal examinations
- Ensure that Pap tests meet quality standards
- Ensure that mammograms meet quality standards
- Reduce deaths due to cancer of the oral cavity and pharynx

Priority Area: *Diabetes and Chronic Disabling Conditions*—Text Chapter 6

Year 2000 Objectives

- Increase years of a healthy life
- Reduce disability from chronic conditions
- Preserve independent functioning in older adults
- Reduce activity limitation from asthma
- Reduce activity limitation due to chronic back conditions
- Reduce hearing impairment
- Reduce visual impairment
- Reduce mental retardation
- Reduce diabetes-related deaths
- Reduce diabetes-related complications
- Reduce diabetes incidence/prevalence
- Reduce prevalence of overweight
- Increase moderate physical activity
- Increase patient education
- Improve clinical assessment of childhood development
- Increase early detection of hearing impairments of children
- Improve clinician assessment of independent functioning in older adults
- Increase counseling about estrogen replacement therapy
- Increase employment of people with disabilities
- Improve service systems for children with or at risk of chronic and disabling conditions
- Reduce prevalence of peptic ulcer disease by preventing its recurrence

- Develop and implement a national process to identify gaps in the Nation's disease prevention and health promotion data
- Increase annual dilated eye exam for people with diabetes

Priority Area: *Substance Abuse: Alcohol and Other Drugs*—Text Chapter 7

Year 2000 Objectives

- Reduce alcohol-related motor vehicle crash deaths
- Reduce cirrhosis deaths
- Reduce drug-related deaths
- Reduce drug abuse-related hospital emergency visits
- Increase the average age of first use of cigarettes, alcohol, and marijuana
- Reduce alcohol, marijuana, and cocaine use by youth
- Reduce heavy drinking by youth
- Reduce overall alcohol consumption
- Increase social disapproval of alcohol, marijuana, and cocaine by youth
- Increase awareness of the harmful effects of addictive substances
- Reduce use of anabolic steroids
- Establish better access to treatment
- Provide alcohol and drug education in schools
- Adopt worksite alcohol/drug policies
- Extend laws related to driving under the influence of intoxicants
- Reduce minors' access to alcohol
- Increase restrictions on promotion of alcohol to youth
- Extend legal blood alcohol concentration tolerance levels
- Increase screening, counseling, and referral by clinicians for alcohol/drug problems
- Increase the number of States with Hospitality Resource Panels

Priority Area: *Tobacco*—Text Chapter 7

Year 2000 Objectives

- Reduce coronary heart disease deaths
- Slow the rise in lung cancer deaths

- Slow the rise in chronic obstructive pulmonary disease deaths
- Reduce cigarette smoking
- Reduce initiation of cigarette smoking by children and youth
- Increase smoking cessation
- Increase smoking cessation during pregnancy
- Reduce child exposure to tobacco smoke at home
- Reduce smokeless tobacco use
- Establish tobacco use prevention programs in schools
- Increase restrictive smoking policies at worksites
- Enact clean indoor air laws
- Enact and enforce laws prohibiting the sale of tobacco products to minors
- Increase States with plans to reduce tobacco use
- Eliminate or restrict tobacco advertising and promotion to youth
- Increase smoking cessation counseling and follow-up by providers
- Reduce oral cavity and pharynx cancers
- Reduce stroke deaths
- Increase average age of first use of cigarettes, alcohol, and marijuana
- Reduce past month substance abuse among young people
- Increase proportion of high school seniors who disapprove of substance use
- Increase the proportion of high school seniors who associate physical or psychological harm with substance use
- Increase the average tobacco excise tax
- Increase proportion of health plans offering treatment for nicotine addiction
- Reduce the number of States with preemptive clean indoor air laws
- Enact laws banning youth access to cigarette vending machines

Priority Area: *Nutrition*—Text Chapter 8

Year 2000 Objectives

- Reduce coronary heart disease deaths

- Reverse the rise in cancer deaths
- Reduce overweight prevalence
- Reduce growth retardation
- Reduce dietary fat intake
- Increase complex carbohydrate and fiber-containing foods
- Increase sound weight loss practices
- Increase calcium intake
- Decrease salt and sodium intake
- Reduce iron deficiency
- Increase breastfeeding
- Decrease baby bottle tooth decay
- Increase use of food labels
- Achieve useful nutrition labeling
- Increase availability of low-fat foods
- Increase low-fat, low-calorie food choices
- Increase school and child care menus consistent with the Dietary Guidelines
- Increase home-delivered meals
- Increase nutrition education in schools
- Increase nutrition education and weight management programs at worksites
- Increase nutrition assessment, counseling, and referrals
- Reduce stroke death
- Reduce colorectal cancer death
- Reduce diabetes incidence/prevalence
- Reduce prevalence of high blood cholesterol
- Increase blood pressure screening
- Reduce adult mean serum cholesterol

Summary

Health is "a state of complete physical, mental, and social well-being not merely the absence of disease or infirmity" according to The World Health Organization. By definition, health is a universal trait. Due to the fact that personal behaviors are one of the four major factors that influence a person's lifespan and quality of life, health also takes on a very individual and unique quality.

The idea of wellness is an individual based approach to health. Wellness is grounded in behavior modification strategies that result in the adoption of low-risk, health enhancing behaviors. By balancing the five components of wellness; emotional, mental,

Figure 1.2
How to Use Healthy Behaviors and Healthy Decision Making to Add Years to Your Life

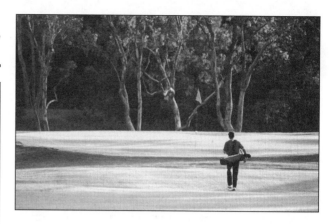

Researchers at the Human Population Laboratory of the California Department of Health published the following list of health related behaviors that have been associated with good health and a long life. These behaviors include:

1. Regular exercise
2. Adequate sleep
3. A good breakfast
4. Regular meals
5. Weight control
6. Abstinence from smoking and drugs
7. Moderate use of (or abstinence from) alcohol

It was shown that by following six of the seven listed behaviors not only is an individual's quality of life greatly improved, but also, men could add 11 years to their lives and women could add seven years to their lives.

social, spiritual, and physical, a person can, to some degree, prevent disease and premature death.

Each decade since 1979, *Healthy People 2000* has defined the nation's current health agenda. Through the objectives listed for specific Priority Areas within *Healthy People 2000,* the importance of prevention in promoting wellness is made clear.

References

Breslow, L. and J. Enstrom. 1980. "Persistence of Health Habits and their Relationship to Mortality." *Preventative Medicine,* 9: 469–483.

Corbin, Charles B., and Ruth Lindsay. *Concepts of Physical Fitness.* New York City, New York: McBrown 1994.

Definitions of Health. Webster's Dictionary. http://www.m-w.com/dictionary.htm

Definition of Health. World Health Organization. http://who.int/aboutwho/en/definition.html

Definition of Wellness. American Holistic Health Association. http://ahha.org

Floyd, P., Mims, S., and C. Yelding-Howard. *Personal Health: Perspectives and Lifestyles.* Englewood, CO: Morton Publishing Co. 1998.

Hahn, Dale B., and Wayne A. Payne. *Understanding Your Health.* New York, NY: McGraw-Hill. 1998.

Health Definitions. Center for Disease Control. http://www.cdc.gov/nchs/data/hp2k99.pdf

Hyman, B., et al. *Fitness for Living.* Dubuque, Iowa: Kendall-Hunt Publishing Co., 1999.

Priority Areas. *Healthy People 2000.* http://odphp.osophs.dhhs.gov/pubs/hp2000

Pruitt, B.E. and J. Stein. *Health Styles.* Boston, MA: Allyn & Bacon, 1999.

Activities

In-Class Activities
    Name Calling
    Class Pictures
    How Do You Spell Relief
    What's in a Name
    You're My Type

Out-of-Class Activities
What's My Line	(1 point)
I Like That	(1 point)
Stress Journal	(2 points)
Have A Laugh	(2 points)
College Schedule of Recent Experience	(2 points)

All activities found within the text.

■ Name Calling

Concept/Description: This activity is an ice breaker designed to get to know class members.

Objective: Remember each class member's name and something about him or her.

Materials: None

Directions:
1. Divide the class into two (or more) large circles.
2. Starting with a volunteer and moving clockwise, have one person introduce him- or herself, then say one thing he or she enjoys doing. For example, "My name is Pat and I play lacrosse."
3. The next person would repeat what Pat said, then add his or her own introduction.
4. Allow group members to help if someone starts to struggle with remembering names.
5. Continue until all class members have been introduced.

■ Class Pictures

Concept/Description: In groups, one member will draw pictures while the other group members try to guess a key word or phrase.

Objective: Be the first group to guess the key word or phrase.

Materials: Draw This cards
Paper
Pens or pencils
Chalkboard
Chalk

Directions:

1. Divide the class into groups of five or six and give each group some scrap paper. Each group needs pens or pencils.
2. Each member of the group counts off.
3. The teacher sits in the center of the room and when ready, asks all the students numbered one to come look at one of the Draw This cards.
4. Students then quickly return to their seats and begin drawing clues so the group members can guess the word or phrase that was on the teacher's card. Note: No words, letters, or numbers may be drawn. No talking is permitted by the person drawing.
5. Group members try to guess what the picture is. They call out their guesses until one is correct or until another group guesses first.
6. The first group to get the correct answer is the winner of the round, and that group receives one point.
7. Keep score on the chalkboard.
8. Continue playing by calling up student two, then three, and so on until everyone has had a chance to draw.
9. The team with the most points is the winner.

"DRAW THIS" Cards

a wedding	shopping
kissing	going to the movies
an argument	fast food
a baby crying	talking on the phone
a person listening	arguing with parents
a fist fight	best friends

"DRAW THIS" Cards (Make Your Own)

NAME _____   SECTION _____   DATE _____

■ How Do You Spell Relief?

Directions: Listed below are some examples of how people deal with stress. With a partner, brainstorm all the ways that people could deal with stress. Include both positive and negative methods. When you have compiled a list, go back and place an X in the boxes of the methods that are healthy ways to deal with stress.

☐ smoking _____   ☐ _____

☐ drinking alcohol _____   ☐ _____

☒ exercise _____   ☐ _____

☐ _____   ☐ _____

☐ _____   ☐ _____

☐ _____   ☐ _____

☐ _____   ☐ _____

☐ _____   ☐ _____

☐ _____   ☐ _____

☐ _____   ☐ _____

☐ _____   ☐ _____

☐ _____   ☐ _____

☐ _____   ☐ _____

From *Just for the Health of It: Unit 5, Stress Management and Self-Esteem Activities* by Patricia Rizzo Toner. Copyright © 1993. Reprinted by permission of Center for Applied Research in Education/Prentice Hall Direct.

■ What's in a Name?

Directions: Write your first and last name vertically in the space provided. Use the letters to write words that describe your positive qualities. Compare yours to your classmates. An example is given below.

P	**atient**
A	**ccepting**
T	**rustworthy**
S	**ociable**
M	**ellow**
I	**ntelligent**
T	**reats people with respect**
H	**umorous**

Try your name below:

■ You're My Type

Directions: Read the explanations of the two personality types below, then take the test to determine which type you are.

Type A Personality

The Type A person is very competitive, often impatient, and feels that he or she must be successful. This person is aggressive and driven to work hard. They often feel that time is of the essence and, therefore, move and talk rapidly. Type A persons are usually impatient listeners. Because they are so driven, Type A persons are more at risk and susceptible to coronary heart disease and other stress-related diseases.

Type B Personality

The Type B person is more laid back and less hurried. This person is usually patient, noncompetitive, and nonaggressive.

Which Type Are You?

Directions: Place a + in the blank if the statement describes you and a − if it does not.

a +   1. I become angry or aggravated if I have to stand in line for more than 10–15 minutes.

a +   2. I try to do more than one thing at a time.

a +   3. I try very hard to win while playing sports or games.

a −   4. I feel guilty if I am doing nothing.

a −   5. I hate to lose and become angry at myself or others if I do.

a +   6. I speak, eat, and move quickly.

a −   7. I interrupt people who talk slowly in order to speed things up.

a +   8. I work better under pressure.

a +   9. I have a strong need to be successful.

a −   10. I set deadlines and schedules for myself.

> **SCORING:** If 6–10 statements describe you, you may be a Type A personality. If only a few describe you, you may be a Type B personality. Some people may be a combination depending on the circumstances. It is important that we are aware of ourselves and learn when and how to relax.

■ What's My Line?

Directions: Place an *X* on each line indicating where you rate yourself. In which areas are you satisfied or dissatisfied? What could you do to improve the areas that need improvement?

Total Slob	Neat Freak
Room should be condemned.	Room is spotless…you could eat off the floor.
└─────────────────────┘	
Hot Head	Cool Operator
Gets angry about every little thing.	Takes a great deal to get me angry.
└─────────────────────┘	
Class Clown	Quiet and Reserved
I say things that usually make others laugh.	I rarely tell jokes.
└─────────────────────┘	
Total Jock	Non-Athletic
I love playing sports.	I am not the least bit interested in sports.
└─────────────────────┘	
Optimist	Pessimist
I see the glass half-full.	I see the glass half-empty.
└─────────────────────┘	
Leader	Follower
└─────────────────────┘	
Health Fanatic	Couch Potato
Exercise and healthy foods are a must.	TV and some junk food for me.
└─────────────────────┘	
Chatterbox	All Ears
I love to talk.	I'd rather listen.
└─────────────────────┘	
Gossiper	My Lips Are Sealed
I love to tell "juicy" stories.	I would never spread rumors.
└─────────────────────┘	
Forgiving	Grudge-Holder
I am able to forgive and forget	I hold grudges for years.
└─────────────────────┘	

From *Just for the Health of It: Unit 5, Stress Management and Self-Esteem Activities* by Patricia Rizzo Toner.
Copyright © 1993. Reprinted by permission of Center for Applied Research in Education/Prentice Hall Direct.

■ I Like That!

Directions: In the spaces under "Activity" write down fifteen things you like to do, such as playing basketball, painting, going to the mall, etc. In each column, place an *X* if the heading applies. Then answer the questions at the bottom of the page.

Activity	Costs more than $5	Requires physical activity	Is done outdoors	Is done often	Is done with friends or family

Are most of the activities you enjoy expensive?

How many of the fifteen things you like to do require physical activity?

How many are done primarily outdoors?

Do you get to do the things you enjoy often? If not, why not?

Are most of the things you enjoy done with people or alone?

From *Just for the Health of It: Unit 5, Stress Management and Self-Esteem Activities* by Patricia Rizzo Toner. Copyright © 1993. Reprinted by permission of Center for Applied Research in Education/Prentice Hall Direct.

■ Stress Journal

Directions: To start managing stress, you must first recognize it. Fill in the stress journal entries twice in the morning, twice in the afternoon, and twice in the evening for two weeks. When the two weeks are over, discuss your observations with your classmates. What causes YOU the most stress? (Use as many sheets as necessary to complete the task.)

Date	Time	Situation	Stress Level	Signs
5/29	9:00 am	(Where? With whom? Doing what?) At work… argued with boss.	(1–100) 85	Heart racing, headache, muscle tension

From *Just for the Health of It: Unit 5, Stress Management and Self-Esteem Activities* by Patricia Rizzo Toner.
Copyright © 1993. Reprinted by permission of Center for Applied Research in Education/Prentice Hall Direct.

NAME _____ SECTION _____ DATE _____

■ Have a Laugh!

Directions: One of the best stress relievers is laughter. Spending time with people who make you
laugh is a good way to relax. Answer the questions below and have a laugh!

1. Who is one of the funniest people you know?

2. What is something this person said or did that made you laugh?

3. What is the funniest thing that has *ever* happened to you?

4. Do you like to tell jokes, hear jokes, or both?

5. Who is your favorite comedian?

6. What is your favorite comedy movie?

7. What is your favorite TV show? Is it a comedy?

8. What is your favorite TV commercial? Is it humorous?

9. Do you think you have a good sense of humor?

10. Did anything make you laugh today? If so, what?

From *Just for the Health of It: Unit 5, Stress Management and Self-Esteem Activities* by Patricia Rizzo Toner.
Copyright © 1993. Reprinted by permission of Center for Applied Research in Education/Prentice Hall Direct.

■ College Schedule of Recent Experience

Purpose   To predict your chances of developing a stress-related illness.

Procedure   On the answer sheet on the following page, indicate the number of times during the last 12 months that each of the following life-change events has happened to you.

1. Entered college.
2. Married.
3. Had either a lot more or a lot less trouble with your boss.
4. Held a job while attending school.
5. Experienced the death of a spouse.
6. Experienced a major change in sleeping habits (sleeping a lot more or a lot less or a change in part of the day when asleep).
7. Experienced the death of a close family member.
8. Experienced a major change in eating habits (a lot more or a lot less food intake or very different meal hours or surroundings).
9. Made a change in or choice of a major field of study.
10. Had a revision of your personal habits (friends, dress, manners, associations).
11. Experienced the death of a close friend.
12. Have been found guilty of minor violations of the law (traffic tickets, jaywalking, etc.).
13. Had an outstanding personal achievement.
14. Experienced pregnancy or fathered a pregnancy.
15. Had a major change in the health or behavior of a family member.
16. Had sexual difficulties.
17. Had trouble with in-laws.
18. Had a major change in the number of family get-togethers (a lot more or a lot less).
19. Had a major change in financial state (a lot worse off or a lot better off than usual).
20. Gained a new family member (through birth, adoption, older person moving in, etc.).
21. Changed your residence or living conditions.
22. Had a major conflict in or change in values.
23. Had a major change in church activities (a lot more or a lot less than usual).
24. Had a marital reconciliation with your mate.
25. Were fired from work.
26. Were divorced.
27. Changed to different line of work.
28. Had a major change in the number or arguments with spouse (either a lot more or a lot less than usual).
29. Had a major change in responsibilities at work (promotion, demotion, lateral transfer).
30. Had your spouse begin or cease work outside the home.
31. Had a marital separation from your mate.
32. Had a major change in the usual type and/or amount of recreation.
33. Had a major change in the use of drugs (a lot more or a lot less).
34. Took a mortgage or loan *less* than $10,000 (such as purchase of a car, TV, school loan, etc.).
35. Had a major personal injury or illness.
36. Had a major change in the use of alcohol (a lot more or a lot less).
37. Had a major change in social activities.
38. Had a major change in the amount of participation in school activities.
39. Had a major change in the amount of independence and responsibility (e.g., for budgeting time).
40. Took a trip or a vacation.
41. Were engaged to be married.
42. Changed to a new school.

43. Changed dating habits.
44. Had trouble with school administration (instructors, advisors, class scheduling, etc.).
45. Broke or had broken a marital engagement or a steady relationship.
46. Had a major change in self-concept or self-awareness.

Answer and Scoring Sheet

First, for the number corresponding to each of the life events listed, indicate the number of times (1, 2, 3, etc.) that the particular event has occurred in your life during the past 12 months. Then multiply each item by the indicated weight, and total the scores.

1. _____	× 50 = _____		24. _____	× 58 = _____	
2. _____	× 77 = _____		25. _____	× 62 = _____	
3. _____	× 38 = _____		26. _____	× 76 = _____	
4. _____	× 43 = _____		27. _____	× 50 = _____	
5. _____	× 87 = _____		28. _____	× 50 = _____	
6. _____	× 34 = _____		29. _____	× 47 = _____	
7. _____	× 77 = _____		30. _____	× 41 = _____	
8. _____	× 30 = _____		31. _____	× 74 = _____	
9. _____	× 41 = _____		32. _____	× 37 = _____	
10. _____	× 45 = _____		33. _____	× 52 = _____	
11. _____	× 68 = _____		34. _____	× 52 = _____	
12. _____	× 22 = _____		35. _____	× 65 = _____	
13. _____	× 40 = _____		36. _____	× 46 = _____	
14. _____	× 68 = _____		37. _____	× 43 = _____	
15. _____	× 56 = _____		38. _____	× 38 = _____	
16. _____	× 58 = _____		39. _____	× 49 = _____	
17. _____	× 42 = _____		40. _____	× 33 = _____	
18. _____	× 26 = _____		41. _____	× 54 = _____	
19. _____	× 53 = _____		42. _____	× 50 = _____	
20. _____	× 50 = _____		43. _____	× 41 = _____	
21. _____	× 42 = _____		44. _____	× 44 = _____	
22. _____	× 50 = _____		45. _____	× 60 = _____	
23. _____	× 36 = _____		46. _____	× 57 = _____	

Subtotal = _____   Subtotal = _____

Total life-change score = _____

Interpretation   The number of life changes that a person experiences each year may be classified as mild, moderate, or excessive. An increased number of life changes is associated with an increase in the incidence of illness and accidents during the following 12-month period. It is estimated that people experiencing only mild life changes over the past year have an estimated 30% chance of becoming ill or having an accident. Those having an excessive number of life changes are at a much higher risk of developing significant health problems. The higher the score in life-change units, the greater the potential for significant illness or accident.

Category	Scoring range
Mild	0–499
Moderate	500–999
Excessive	1000 or above

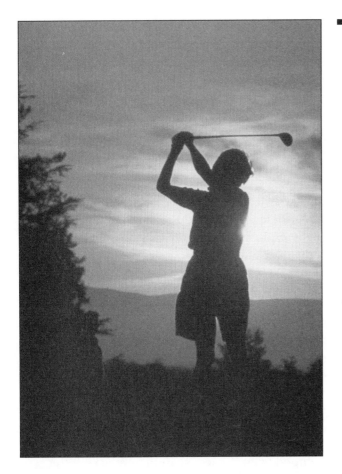

Chapter Two

Cardiovascular and Muscular Fitness

"You must have long-range goals to keep you from being frustrated by short-range failures."

—Charles C. Noble

OBJECTIVES

Students will be able to:

- Define key terms related to cardiovascular and muscular fitness.

- Explain how exercise improves the function of the heart and vascular system.

- Explain the relationship between cardiovascular fitness and heart disease.

- Be able to determine aerobic threshold of training, target heart rate zones, and FITT formula components.

- Identify techniques used to measure cardiovascular fitness.

- Identify the benefits of resistance training.

- Understand the physiological adaptations of resistance training.

- Understand how to design a resistance training program for beginners.

The purpose of this chapter is to present the basic components of cardiovascular and muscular fitness. Cardiovascular fitness is often referred to as the most important aspect of physical fitness because of its relevance to good health and optimal performance. Muscular fitness is important because of its effect on efficiency of human movement and basal metabolic rate.

Defining Physical Fitness

As stated in chapter one, physical activity and fitness are important components of health as defined by Healthy People 2000: National Health Promotion and Disease Prevention. There are two types of physical fitness: health-related fitness and skill-related fitness. *Health-related fitness* consists of cardiovascular fitness, muscular strength and endurance, flexibility, and optimal body composition. The components of health-related fitness affect the body's ability to function efficiently and effectively. Optimal health-related fitness is not possible without regular, appropriately designed exercise. Most health clubs and fitness classes focus primarily on the health-related fitness components. *Skill-related fitness* includes agility, balance, coordination, reaction time, speed, and power. Skill related fitness is not essential in order to have cardiovascular fitness nor will it necessarily make a person healthier. However, all physical activities are performed with greater efficiency when the skill-related fitness components are increased because the activities require less energy.

The health-related fitness component of *cardiovascular fitness* refers to the ability of the heart, lungs, circulatory system, and energy supply system to perform at optimum levels for extended periods of time. The term cardiovascular endurance is interchangeable with cardiovascular fitness. *Cardiovascular endurance* is defined as the ability of the body to perform prolonged, large-muscle, dynamic exercise at moderate to high levels of intensity. The word *aerobic* means in the presence of oxygen and is used synonymously with cardiovascular when describing a type of exercise. Thus, exercise designed to provide cardiovascular fitness or cardiovascular endurance can be described as cardiovascular or aerobic. How important is participation in physical activity in achieving and maintaining good health?

Since 1992, the American Heart Association has considered the lack of physical activity as important a risk factor for heart disease as high blood cholesterol, high blood pressure, and cigarette smoking. According to the American Heart Association 1998 statistics, almost 59 million Americans have one or more forms of cardiovascular disease, about one-sixth of all people killed by cardiovascular disease are under the age of 65, and coronary heart disease is the single leading cause of death in America today. The U.S. Centers for Disease Control and Prevention and the American College of Sports Medicine reported that 250,00 lives are lost each year due to inactivity (Pate et al., 1995). In 1996 the U.S. Surgeon General's Report made several definitive statements regarding physical activity and its impact on one's health. The following conclusions were stated in the report:

1. people of all ages, both male and female, benefit from regular physical activity;
2. significant health benefits can be obtained by moderately increasing daily activity on most, if not all, days of the week;
3. additional health benefits can be gained through greater amounts of physical activity;

4. physical activity reduces the risk of premature mortality in general, and of coronary heart disease, hypertension, colon cancer, and diabetes mellitus in particular;
5. more than 60 percent of American adults are not regularly physically active; and
6. nearly half of American youth 12 to 21 years of age are not vigorously active on a regular basis.

The American Heart Association and the Centers for Disease Control and Prevention websites listed at the end of this chapter will provide current information and statistics.

As we realize there are many negative effects associated with lack of activity, it is important to realize the many potential benefits associated with aerobic exercise, as well—specifically with aerobic fitness. When one is aerobically fit, there is an overall reduction in the risk of coronary artery disease, i.e., stroke, blood vessel diseases, and heart diseases. Related to this reduction, there is a decrease in resting heart rate due to the improved efficiency of the heart. There is also an increase in *stroke volume*, which is the amount of blood pumped from the left or right ventricle with each heartbeat. A decrease in *systolic blood pressure*, which is the highest arterial blood pressure attained during the heart cycle, and a decrease in the *diastolic blood pressure*, or lowest arterial pressure attained during the heart cycle, also occurs. There is also an increase in *collateral circulation*, which refers to the number of functioning capillaries both in the heart and throughout the body. In addition to the specific physiological changes just listed, other benefits of a mental, emotional, and physical nature will increase with regular aerobic exercise. Some of the potential benefits that have been documented when aerobic fitness levels increase are: a decrease in percent body fat, an increase in strength of connective tissues, a reduction in mental anxiety and depression, along with improved sleep patterns, a decrease in the speed of the aging process, an improvement in stress management, and an increase in cognitive abilities (Sharkey, 1997).

The Cardiovascular System

It is important to understand the function of the heart in any discussion of cardiovascular fitness.

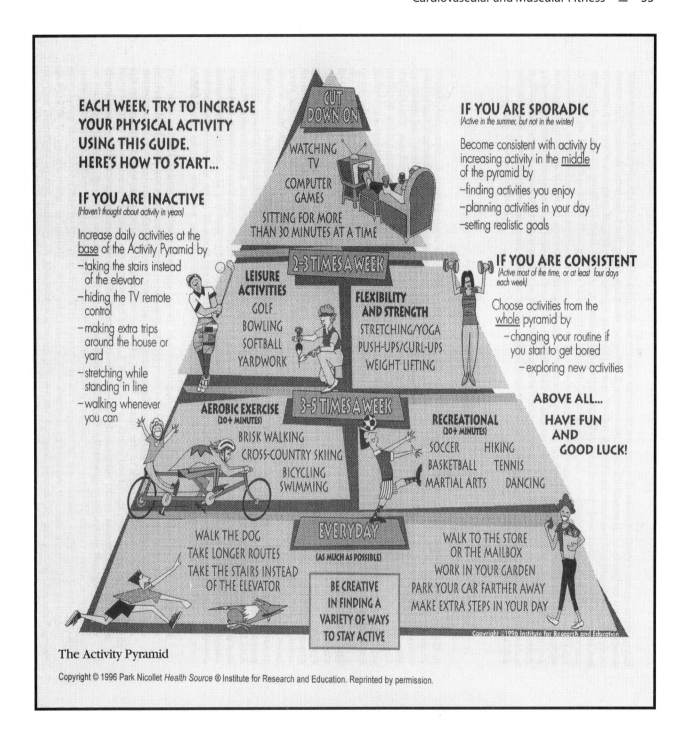

The Activity Pyramid

EACH WEEK, TRY TO INCREASE YOUR PHYSICAL ACTIVITY USING THIS GUIDE. HERE'S HOW TO START...

IF YOU ARE INACTIVE
(Haven't thought about activity in years)

Increase daily activities at the base of the Activity Pyramid by
- taking the stairs instead of the elevator
- hiding the TV remote control
- making extra trips around the house or yard
- stretching while standing in line
- walking whenever you can

IF YOU ARE SPORADIC
(Active in the summer, but not in the winter)

Become consistent with activity by increasing activity in the middle of the pyramid by
- finding activities you enjoy
- planning activities in your day
- setting realistic goals

IF YOU ARE CONSISTENT
(Active most of the time, or at least four days each week)

Choose activities from the whole pyramid by
- changing your routine if you start to get bored
- exploring new activities

ABOVE ALL...
HAVE FUN AND GOOD LUCK!

CUT DOWN ON
WATCHING TV
COMPUTER GAMES
SITTING FOR MORE THAN 30 MINUTES AT A TIME

2-3 TIMES A WEEK

LEISURE ACTIVITIES
GOLF
BOWLING
SOFTBALL
YARDWORK

FLEXIBILITY AND STRENGTH
STRETCHING/YOGA
PUSH-UPS/CURL-UPS
WEIGHT LIFTING

3-5 TIMES A WEEK

AEROBIC EXERCISE (20+ MINUTES)
BRISK WALKING
CROSS-COUNTRY SKIING
BICYCLING
SWIMMING

RECREATIONAL (20+ MINUTES)
SOCCER   HIKING
BASKETBALL   TENNIS
MARTIAL ARTS   DANCING

EVERYDAY
(AS MUCH AS POSSIBLE)

WALK THE DOG
TAKE LONGER ROUTES
TAKE THE STAIRS INSTEAD OF THE ELEVATOR

BE CREATIVE IN FINDING A VARIETY OF WAYS TO STAY ACTIVE

WALK TO THE STORE OR THE MAILBOX
WORK IN YOUR GARDEN
PARK YOUR CAR FARTHER AWAY
MAKE EXTRA STEPS IN YOUR DAY

Copyright ©1996 Institute for Research and Education

A normal cardiac cycle is initiated during activity in the *sinoatrial node*, located in the *right atrium*. The impulse spreads across both the right and left atria causing contraction and continues down to the *atrioventricular node* located between the atria and *ventricles*. The impulse is transmitted to the ventricles through specialized fibers called *Purkinje fibers*, causing the ventricles to contract simultaneously. Blood from the right ventricle goes to the lungs and blood from the left ventricle goes throughout the body.

Heart rate becomes elevated during exercise because of the increase in demand for oxygen in the muscle tissues. Oxygen, attached to hemoglobin molecules, is transported in the blood; therefore the heart pumps at a faster rate to meet the increased demand for oxygen. The heart is a muscle, and like other muscles, it becomes stronger with exercise. Through regular exercise, the heart will increase slightly in size and significantly in strength, which results in an increased stroke volume. The primary difference is seen in the increased thickness and strength of the left ventricle wall. As a result of exercise, blood plasma volume increases, which will also allow stroke volume to increase. These two factors will cause one's resting heart rate to decrease, one's exercising heart rate will become more efficient, and there will be a quicker return to a resting heart rate after exercise ceases. This strengthening of the heart will also allow it to be more efficient when demands are imposed on it through sympathetic nerve stimulation. *Sympathetic nerve stimulation* is responsible for the fight or flight response experienced as a result of emotional or physical stress. High fitness levels decrease the impact of this stress on the heart. Lack of exercise can contribute to many cardiovascular diseases and conditions, including *myocardial infarction*, or heart attack; *angina pectoris*, a condition caused by insufficient blood flow to the heart muscle that results in severe chest pain; and *atherosclerosis*, a thickening and loss of elasticity in the artery walls.

Closely associated with the function and efficiency of the heart is the function and efficiency of the circulatory system. A brief summary of how the circulatory system works is as follows: deoxygenated blood flows from the body into the right atrium through the *superior vena cava, the coronary sinus* and the *inferior vena cava*. It passes through the *tricuspid valve* into the right ventricle, and through the *pulmonary semilunar valve* into the pulmonary artery and the right and left lungs. The blood becomes oxygenated in the lungs and returns to the left atrium via the pulmonary veins. It passes through the *bicuspid valve* into the left ventricle, through the *aortic semilunar valve* to the aorta, then through various arteries to specific destinations in the body. The blood flows from arteries into capillaries where oxygen is released and waste products are collected and removed from the tissues. The deoxygenated blood then makes the return trip to the heart through the venous system. As a result of aerobic exercise, blood flow improves to the skeletal muscles due to an increase in stroke volume, an increase in the number of capillaries, and an increase in the function of existing capillaries. This provides more efficient circulation both during exercise and during daily activities.

Blood flow to the heart muscle is provided by two coronary arteries that branch off from the aorta and form a series of smaller vessels. With regular aerobic activity, the size of the coronary blood vessels increases and collateral circulation improves. These minute blood vessels can supply oxygen to the cardiac muscle tissue when a sudden block occurs in a major vessel, such as during a heart attack. Often the degree of developed collateral circulation, or the extent to which it can be developed, determines one's ability to survive a myocardial infarction, or heart attack. The function of collateral blood vessels increases within a few seconds after a heart attack and again after approximately 24 hours.

The lungs, air passages, and muscles involved in breathing which supply oxygen and remove carbon dioxide from the body are known as the *respiratory system*. Air enters the nose and mouth where it is conformed to body temperature, filtered, and humidified, and flows into the *trachea*. It then passes into the two *bronchi* that branch into each lung. The bronchi branch into smaller *bronchioles* that lead into the *alveolar ducts*. The alveolar ducts are surrounded by the microscopic *alveoli*, which is where gas exchange takes place. During exercise, pulmonary ventilation, which is the movement of gases into and out of the lungs, increases in direct proportion to the body's metabolic needs. At lower exercise intensities, this is accomplished by increases in respiration depth. At higher intensities, the rate of respiration also increases. Although fatigue in strenuous exercise is frequently referred to as feeling "out of breath" or "winded," it appears that the normal capacity for pulmonary ventilation does not limit exercise performance (McArdle, Katch and Katch, 1999). In a normal environment, one inhales sufficient amounts of oxygen. The breathing limitation is in the efficiency of the oxygen exchange at the cellular level. The benefit of aerobic exercise to the respiratory system is primarily in an increase in strength and endurance of the respiratory muscles, not an increase in lung volume. Maximal pulmonary ventilation volumes are dependent on body size (Wilmore and Costill, 1999). Muscles that elevate the thorax are referred to as *muscles of inspiration*. They are the diaphragm, external intercostal muscles, sternocleidomastoids, scapular elevators and anterior serrat, scleni, and spinal erector muscles. *Muscles of expiration*, which depress the thorax, include abdominal muscles, internal intercostal muscles, and posterior inferior serrati. Regular aerobic training will result in an increase in both the strength and endurance of these muscles, and will also result in more efficient respiration.

All human movement is dependent upon a sufficient supply of energy. The source of this energy is the food consumed on a daily basis: fats, proteins, and carbohydrates. However, this food is not transferred directly to the cells for use. Through a series of chemical reactions, food is converted to the high-energy compound *adenosine triphosphate (ATP)*. The energy from the breakdown of this compound allows the cells to perform work. There are three specific energy systems that can provide energy as the ATP compound is broken down. Exercise intensity and duration determines which of the three energy systems is activated. The energy needed for high intensity and short duration activity comes from *creatine phosphate* stored in muscle tissue, which can be used to synthesize ATP and to maintain intense exercise for a short period of time. This energy system, known as the *ATP-PC system*, or immediate system, can be activated very rapidly and depleted very rapidly. The ATP-PC system is used in activities such as hitting a tennis ball, throwing a football, and running a 100-meter dash.

Another energy supplying system that is short term is the *lactic acid* or *glycolytic nonoxidative system*. The energy for this system is supplied from stored muscle glycogen and from anaerobic glycolysis, which results in the accumulation of *lactic acid*. This is what is commonly referred to as anaerobic exercise. This energy system can be relied on to provide energy for one to three minutes during exercise of maximum intensity. The limiting factor in this energy system is the inability to use oxygen efficiently enough to keep up with the energy demand and the accumulation of lactic acid.

A third energy system is the *aerobic* or *oxidative system*, which produces a high-energy yield and is very efficient as long as there is an adequate supply of oxygen at the cellular level. This system can function for a prolonged period of time once

TABLE 2.1. Characteristics of the Body's Energy Systems

	Energy System*		
	Immediate	**Nonoxidative**	**Oxidative**
Duration of activity for which system predominates	0–10 seconds	10 seconds–2 minutes	>2 minutes
Intensity of activity for which system predominates	High	High	Low to moderately high
Rate of ATP production	Immediate, very rapid	Rapid	Slower but prolonged
Fuel	Adenosine triphosphate (ATP), creatine phosphate (CP)	Muscle stores of glycogen and glucose	Body stores of glycogen, glucose, fat, and protein
Oxygen used?	No	No	Yes
Sample activities	Weight lifting, picking up a bag of groceries	400-meter run, running up several flights of stairs	1500-meter run, 30-minute walk, standing in line for a long time

*For most activities, all three systems contribute to energy production; the duration and intensity of the activity determine which system predominates.

SOURCE: Adapted from Brooks, G. A., T. D. Fahey, and T. P. White. 1996. Exercise Physiology: Human Bioenergetics and Its Applications, 2d ed. Mountain View, Calif.: Mayfield.

steady state is achieved, as evidenced by individuals who run in races of 150 miles and more. This energy system responds most to aerobic fitness training and is important in activities with a duration of more than two minutes. All three of these energy systems are activated in orderly progression during one exercise bout. They do not turn off and on like a faucet, but instead, contribute to energy production simultaneously with one being more dominant than the other, depending on the situation. The individual who is highly trained in fitness and aerobic activities will become dependent upon the aerobic energy system quicker and with less oxygen deficiency than the untrained individual. The total oxygen consumed per minute during exercise is much greater for the trained as opposed to the untrained individual. All three systems use carbohydrates as an energy source, but only the aerobic system can use fat as an energy source.

Exercise Prescription for Cardiovascular Fitness

To improve cardiovascular fitness, one must have a well-designed regimen of cardiovascular exercise. In order for improvement to occur, specific guidelines must be adhered to when designing a personal exercise program. As will be discussed later, the following guidelines apply not only to aerobic exercise, but to other components of physical fitness as well. The FITT acronym is easy to remember when identifying an appropriate cardiovascular exercise prescription: frequency, intensity, time and type. The "F" in the FITT formula represents frequency. *Frequency* refers to the number of exercise sessions per week. In order to maintain a level of physical fitness, aerobic exercise must be performed a minimum of two times per week. The American College of Sports Medicine recommends three to five days per week to improve cardiorespiratory fitness (Pollock et al., 1998). For individuals with a low level of aerobic fitness, beginning an exercise program by working out two times a week will result in an initial increase in aerobic fitness level. However, after some time, frequency will need to be increased for improvement to continue. Once a desired fitness level is obtained, aerobic exercise can be safely done on a daily basis.

The second letter in FITT stands for intensity. *Intensity* refers to how hard one is working, and it can be measured by several techniques. These techniques include measuring the heart rate while exercising, rating the perceived exertion, and the talk test. To use heart rate as a measure of intensity, one's target heart rate range needs to be calculated before exercising. Target heart rate range is the intensity of training necessary to achieve cardiovascular improvement. This target heart rate range is a range that indicates what an individual's heart rate should be during exercise. Calculation of target heart rate range is done by multiplying maximum heart rate (220 minus one's age) by a designated percentage. The American College of Sports Medicine guidelines for intensity recommends working between 55 and 90% of maximum heart rate, or between 50 and 85% of heart rate reserve (maximum heart rate minus resting heart rate). For individuals who are very unfit, the recommended range is 55 to 64% of maximum heart rate or 40 to 49% of heart rate reserve (Pollock et al., 1998).

The third factor to be considered when designing a cardiovascular exercise workout is time, or duration. The first "T" in the FITT formula refers to the *time* or length of each exercise session. For benefits to be accrued in the cardiovascular system, exercise duration should be a minimum of 20 minutes of continuous exercise or several intermittent exercise sessions of a minimum of 10 minutes each. Some beginning exercisers may not be capable of exercising continuously for 20 minutes at a prescribed intensity. While a minimum of 20 minutes is recommended, a duration of 10 minutes can certainly be beneficial to people who are at a low fitness level and just beginning an exercise program. Duration and exercise intensity are interdependent. For the nonathlete who is attempting to increase aerobic fitness, exercise intensity should decrease as duration increases, and as duration decreases, exercise intensity can increase. Exercise intensity levels should remain within recommended guidelines, while maximum duration is only limited by the participant's available fuel for energy and mental determination to keep going.

Another factor that should be considered in determining a cardiovascular exercise prescription is *type*, or mode, of exercise. Type of exercise represents the final "T" in FITT. The choice of exercise modality is up to each individual, but one must keep in mind the specific requirements of cardiovascular exercise: use the large muscle groups via continuous and rhythmic movement, and exercise for a duration of 20 minutes or more in the target heart rate range a minimum of three times per week. Common types of aerobic exercise include running, walking, swimming, step aerobics, cross-country skiing, biking, or using a machine such as a rower, stairstepper, or treadmill. However, these are certainly not the only types of exercise available. Any exercise that meets the requirements of intensity and duration is acceptable. Some sports can provide aerobic exercise, depending on the nature of the sport, the position being played, and the skill level of the player. For example, an indoor soccer player could get an aerobic workout by playing a game, provided there is constant movement and training heart rate was maintained in the target heart rate range. Many sports provide an excellent way for people to expend a lot of energy and burn a significant number of calories, but the sports' play some and rest some nature prevents them from being aerobic exercise.

A good cardiovascular workout follows a specific sequence of events. First and foremost, to prepare the body and increase the comfort level for a cardiovascular workout, a warm-up is crucial. The purpose of the warm-up is to prepare the body for the more vigorous work to come. More specifically, the warm-up should increase body temperature, increase heart rate, increase blood flow to the muscles that will be used during the workout, and include some rhythmic movement to loosen muscles that may be cold and/or tight. A warm-up should raise the pulse from a resting rate to a rate somewhere near the low end of the recommended heart rate training zone. Beginning vigorous exercise without some kind of warm-up is not only difficult physically and mentally, but it can also contribute to musculoskeletal injuries. It is important to warm up and stretch specifically the muscles that will be used during the workout. For example, if the aerobic workout is lap swimming for 30 minutes, the upper body would need to be stretched more than if the workout were a 30-minute run. After an aerobic exercise session, the heart rate should be lowered gradually by slowly lowering the intensity of the exercise. Sudden stops are not recommended and can lead to muscle cramps. After a gradual cool-down, often walking, static stretching of the appropriate muscle groups is needed and highly recommended. To review, the sequence of a cardiovascular workout should be as follows: warm-up, stretch, workout, cool down, stretch again.

Principles of Cardiovascular Fitness Training

There are specific principles that can be applied to any exercise program. The focus for this discussion will be cardiovascular fitness. A later discussion will include muscular strength and endurance. The concept of *overload and adaptation* is important in understanding how the body responds to exercise. The principle of overload and adaptation states that in order for a body system to become more efficient or stronger, it must be stressed beyond its normal working level. In other words, it must be overloaded. When this overload occurs, the body system will respond by eventually adapting to this new load and increasing its work efficiency until another plateau is reached. When this occurs, another overload must be applied for another gain to be accomplished. The cardiovascular system can be overloaded in more than one way. For example, a person has been running for a few months and is running a distance of three miles in 30 minutes. The runner never goes farther than three miles and never runs faster than a 10-minute per mile pace. For this individual, some techniques of overloading would be: to increase distance, to run the same distance at a faster pace, or to add hills or sprint segments to the run. The principle of overload and adaptation applies to muscular strength, endurance, and flexibility training, as well, and will be referred to later in a discussion on these topics.

The *principle of specificity* refers to training specifically for an activity, or isolating a specific muscle group and/or movement pattern one would like to improve. For example, a 200-meter sprinter would not train by running long, slow distance. Likewise, a racewalker would not train for competition by swimming. Workouts must be specific to one's goal with respect to the type of exercise, intensity, and duration. *Cross training*, defined as using several different types of training, has recently increased in popularity. The benefits of cross training are to prevent injury from over use and to decrease boredom. The principle of specificity does not negate participation in cross training activities; rather, it indicates that the primary training protocol should be in one's chosen activity.

The *principle of individual differences* states that individuals will respond differently to the same training protocol. This difference in response is primarily the result of different fitness levels at the beginning of the training process. Age, gender, and genetic composition, will also cause individual responses to specific activities to differ. Coaches, athletic trainers, and personal trainers should be especially aware of this principle when designing workouts in order to achieve maximum performance levels.

The inevitable process of losing cardiovascular benefits with cessation of aerobic activity is known as the *reversibility principle*. Physiological changes will occur within the first two weeks of detraining and will continue for several months. Bed rest causes this detraining process to greatly accelerate. The reversibility principle is clearly the justification for off-season programs for athletes and immediate initiation of physical rehabilitation programs for individuals with limited mobility.

Evaluation of Cardiovascular Fitness

There are many ways to measure one's level of cardiovascular fitness. One of the more precise ways, which is often used in hospital or research laboratory settings, is a $VO_{2\,max}$ test, or exercise stress test. The $VO_{2\,max}$ test measures maximal oxygen uptake by analyzing expired air of an individual performing exercise of progressing intensity. The rate of work increases until the $VO_{2\,max}$ no longer increases. This test can be performed on a treadmill, a bicycle ergometer, or by performing a series of steps on an elevated surface. This test requires special training and knowledge by the administrator, and can require expensive equipment to perform. Other ways to measure cardiovascular fitness include the 1.5-mile run, 1.5-mile walk, 12-minute run, 1-mile walk, and various submaximal tests on cycle ergometers and treadmills. Research has been done using these tests to develop norms and standards for different age groups and genders making them reliable for use outside the laboratory setting with minimal training for the test administrator.

Another technique for measuring exercise intensity is through self-evaluation of how hard one is working. Gunner Borg designed the *Rating of Perceived Exertion Scale* in the early 1950s. It is a numbered scale from 6 to 20, with the lowest numbers being "very, very light" exercise and the highest numbers being "maximal" exercise, and the numbers in between representing a gradual increase in difficulty in exercise intensity, from low to high.

Using this scale, a rating of 10 corresponds roughly to 50% of maximal heart rate and a rating of 16 corresponds roughly to 90% of maximal heart rate. This scale is a useful tool for estimating exercise intensity when exact measures are not needed, and it is often used in fitness classes and health clubs.

A third, and probably the easiest, technique to measure exercise intensity is the *talk test*. If one is exercising and must laboriously breath rather than participate in a conversation, the exercise intensity is too high and training heart rate has probably been exceeded. Exercise at this intensity will be difficult to maintain for long periods of time. On the other hand, if one is able to sing, intensity level is probably insufficient for improvement in one's fitness level.

A *recovery heart rate* is also a good indicator of one's level of cardiovascular fitness. Recovery heart rate is taken after an exercise session is completed typically for 30 seconds and multiplied by two for a per minute count. The higher a person's level of cardiovascular fitness, the less time it will take after exercise for the heart rate to return to a pre-exercise level. One minute after the cessation of exercise, a male heart rate should have returned to below 90, and a female heart rate to below 100, beats per minute. Five minutes post exercise, both male and female heart rates should be below 80 beats per minute. This is an indication not only of one's fitness level, but also of the adequacy of a cool-down period.

Related Topics

Although injuries do occur during exercise, the benefits of regular exercise far outweigh the risk of injury. In most cases, proper training, clothing and equipment will prevent injuries. Some common injuries resulting from exercise include joint sprains, muscle strains, and other musculoskeletal problems. Weight-bearing forms of exercise will obviously cause more stress on the joints, but also have benefits that non-weight-bearing activities do not have, such as increasing strength of the bones and other connective tissues. Avoiding injury requires common sense and moderation. One should not attempt to self-diagnose, nor try to "train through the pain." Pain is a signal that something is wrong, and activity should be stopped until the source of the pain is identified and a trained medical person gives permission to begin again. Of course, using proper equipment, wearing proper clothing and shoes, and practicing correct technique are essential for injury prevention. Remember also to take into consideration environmental conditions such as temperature, air pollution, wind-chill, altitude and humidity that can affect one's health and safety. Use common sense when environmental conditions are significant!

The internal conditions of the body before and during exercise are even more crucial than exercising with the proper external conditions. Eating immediately before exercising will usually result in poor performance, stomach cramps and sometimes even vomiting. Eating should take place at least two hours prior to exercise for maximum comfort. The type of food consumed on a daily basis is an important factor to consider when developing cardiovascular fitness, and especially when training for competitive events. The recommendations for individuals involved in a regular exercise program are: 55 to 60% of total calories consumed should be from carbohydrates, 25 to 30% from fat, and 12 to 15% from protein. Individuals who are involved in a high-intensity training program should consume a higher amount of protein and less fat for muscle growth and maintenance.

Proper hydration is also necessary for the body to function properly. Water aids in controlling body temperature, contributes to the structure and form of the body, and provides the liquid environment for cell processes. When the thirst mechanism is activated, dehydration has already begun. It is important to pre-hydrate, drink before thirst occurs, and especially drink before exercising. The standard recommendation is to drink at least six 8-ounce glasses of water a day. Exercise increases the body's demand for water due to an increase in metabolic rate and body temperature. Therefore, this amount should be increased. Drinking water every waking hour is a good habit for individuals who exercise on a regular basis. Before, during, and after aerobic exercise, increase the amount of water consumed. Water is necessary for the efficient functioning of the body; thus, the importance of hydration cannot be over stated. Electrolyte levels, especially calcium, sodium and potassium, are critically important in muscle contraction and should also be carefully maintained. This may be accomplished through re-hydrating with sport drinks.

The focus of this discussion has been on aerobic fitness. However, anaerobic conditioning is also important. The common definition for the word anaerobic is "in the absence of oxygen." This is not an accurate definition, however, because all exercise is performed in the presence of oxygen. *Anaerobic exercise* is exercise performed at intensity levels so great that the body's demand for oxygen exceeds its ability to supply it. Anaerobic exercise is especially useful for developing anaerobic fitness; however, it also contributes to the development of cardiovascular fitness. Although it is not recommended for all people, those who are interested in participating in competitive sports should engage in some type of high intensity, anaerobic workout program (Corbin and Lindsey 1994). Compared to aerobic exercise, anaerobic exercise consists of high intensity, short duration, sprint activities, with energy being supplied primarily from carbohydrates. The principles of overload and adaptation and specificity also apply to anaerobic conditioning.

Muscular Fitness

A second component of health related fitness is muscular fitness. Muscular fitness includes two specific components: muscular strength and muscular endurance. *Muscular strength* is the force or tension a muscle or muscle group can exert against a resistance in one maximal effort. *Muscular endurance* is the ability or capacity of a muscle group to perform repeated contractions against a load, or to sustain a contraction for an extended period of time. Muscular fitness focuses on developing skeletal muscle strength and endurance as opposed to developing cardiac or smooth muscle tissue.

Muscle Fiber Types

Skeletal muscle tissue, which attaches to bones and produces all human movement, is characterized by long, cylindrical, multinucleated fibers. These fibers are under voluntary control, with their main function being contraction, which then results in movement. Skeletal muscle fibers are identified as either slow-twitch or fast-twitch, based on characteristics and abilities. Most skeletal muscles contain a combination of both fiber types. The percentage of each fiber type found in individual muscles is genetically determined; however, muscular fitness training or inactivity may cause a slight change in muscle fiber composition. *Slow-twitch fibers* generate small amounts of force, are very resistant to fatigue, and are used primarily in aerobic activity. These aerobic fibers are also known as red, tonic, Type I, and slow oxidative fibers. *Fast-twitch fibers* are capable of generating large amounts of force quickly, but they fatigue very rapidly. Fast-twitch fibers are used in activities that require a burst of speed, such as sprinting from first to second base in baseball. These anaerobic fibers are called white, phasic, Type II, and fast oxidative.

Cardiac and smooth muscle fibers are activated by involuntary neural stimulation. *Cardiac muscle* is striated and contains actin and myosin filaments. The heart is composed of this type of muscle tissue, which responds to cardiovascular training. *Smooth muscle fibers* are found in the walls of blood vessels, intestines, stomach, esophagus and other organs and function to move blood, food, waste products and other body fluids throughout the body. They contain actin and myosin filaments, but are not striated and do not respond to training.

Muscular Contractions

Skeletal muscles are divided into *motor units*, which are defined as the motor nerve and the muscle fibers it innervates. Skeletal muscle fibers are striated with alternating light and dark bands of filaments called *actin* and *myosin*. The actin and myosin filaments are composed of proteins and cause muscle contraction by sliding across each other. This process is known as the *sliding filament theory*. The length of the muscle fiber shortens during contraction, but the lengths of actin and myosin filaments do not change. This contraction process is divided into four phases (Fox et al., 1989):

Rest—Under resting conditions, the cross-bridges of the myosin filaments do not interact with the actin filaments.

Excitation-contraction coupling—An impulse from a motor nerve starts a series of reactions resulting in the coupling of actin and myosin that generates force.

Contraction (tension development)—The formation of actomyosin leads to force development.

Recharging—The bond between myosin and actin is broken (by ATP binding) freeing up the cross-bridge on the myosin filament.

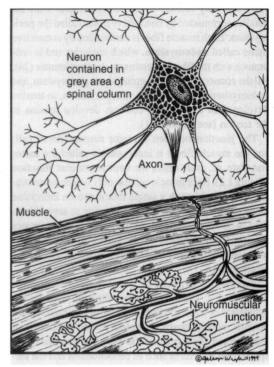

© K. Galasyn-Wright, 1994.

Figure 2.2 A motor unit, consisting of a motor neuron and the muscle fibers it innervates. There are typically many more than three muscle fibers in a single motor unit.

Skeletal muscle contraction is either dynamic or static. Isotonic contraction is one form of dynamic contraction. During *isotonic contraction* the muscle shortens and lengthens during one complete repetition. A contraction in which the muscle is shortening is identified as *concentric contraction*, and a contraction in which the muscle is lengthening is known as *eccentric contraction*. The amount of muscle tension required to move an object through a complete range of motion will vary, while the amount of outside resistance remains the same. Lifting free weights is the most common example of isotonic contraction for muscular fitness.

Isokinetic contractions are also dynamic contractions. They are contractions that are concentric only, performed on calibrated machines that require maximal muscle tension throughout the entire range of motion at a sustained speed. The amount of external resistance varies as the movement is performed. The advantage of isokinetic exercise is that a level very close to maximal force is required throughout the entire movement. The argument can be made that exerting maximal muscle

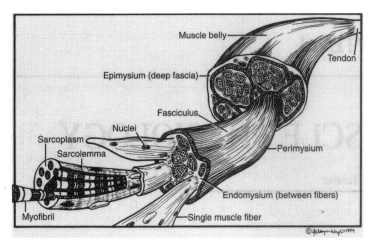

Figure 2.3 Schematic drawing of a muscle illustrating three types of connective tissue: epimysium (the outer layer), perimysium (surrounding each fasciculus, or group of fibers), and endomysium (surrounding individual fibers).

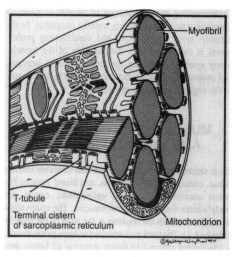

Figure 2.4 Sectional view of a muscle fiber.

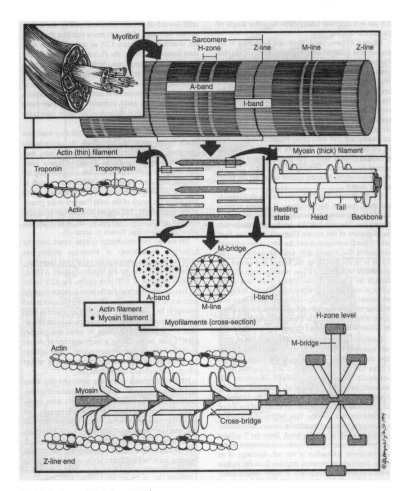

Figure 2.5 Detailed view of the myosin and actin protein filaments in muscle. The arrangement of myosin (thick) and actin (thin) filaments gives skeletal muscle its striated appearance.

tension throughout the entire range of motion will cause maximum muscle development. Another type of dynamic resistance training that is used by individuals who desire very specific and very powerful muscular development is *plyometric training*. This type of training uses the stretch-recoil ability of skeletal muscle, and implements a jumping motion with each exercise. Athletes and individuals who desire maximum performance incorporate plyometric activities into their training protocols.

Static or *isometric contractions* develop tension with no change in length of the muscle. An example of an isometric exercise is pushing against an immovable object, or pushing one's right arm against one's stationary left arm. Isometric contractions cause a rapid increase in muscle strength, but are limited to the joint angle used during training. Isometric training works well for rehabilitation purposes, but is limited in determining the appropriate force to be applied because measurements of isometric force require specific equipment.

Regardless of the type of resistance training used, the amount of force a particular muscle can produce at any point in time is determined by several variables. According to Wilmore and Costill (1999), the development of muscle force is dependent upon the following: the number of motor units activated, the type of motor units activated, the size of the muscle, the muscle's initial length when activated, the angle of the joint, and the muscle's speed of action.

Benefits of Muscular Fitness

Several physiological adaptations occur as a result of resistance training. Strength gains can be seen within the first six weeks, with little or no change in muscle size, and are attributed to neural changes. These changes include decreased activation of antagonistic muscles, learning how to perform the activity, changes in activation of the motor unit, improved recruitment patterns of muscle fibers, change in the gain of the muscle spindle and Golgi tendon organ, and reduction in the sensitivity of force-producing limiting factors.

As strength training activities continue, *hypertrophy*, or an increase in the size of the muscle fibers, occurs. To a limited extent *hyperplasia*, or an increase in the number of fibers, may also occur with continued training. Another result from training is an increase in the amount of energy available for contraction. Carbohydrates are stored in the form of glycogen in the muscle and can be used as the primary energy source for contraction. These muscle glycogen stores increase as a result of training. Bone and connective tissue also undergo changes with resistance training, including an increase in bone matrix, an increase in bone mineral density, and an increase in mass and tensile strength of ligaments and tendons. These increases help prevent injury and decrease the chance of development of osteoporosis after middle age.

Along with the physiological adaptations previously discussed come benefits that improve the quality of one's life. These benefits of muscular fitness include: an increase in muscular strength, power and endurance, a higher percentage of fat-free body mass, improved posture, increased metabolic rate, improved ease of movement; increased resistance to muscle fatigue, increased strength of tendons, ligaments and bones, decreased risk of low back pain, and increased energy and vitality. A summary of adaptations to muscular fitness training can be found in Table 2.

Principles of Muscular Fitness Training

Just as in cardiovascular training, resistance training should be designed with specific goals in mind. The *principle of specificity*, which refers to training for a specific activity, or isolating the specific muscle groups and/or movement pattern that one would like to improve, must be applied in resistance training. In following the principle of specificity, specific exercises should be selected which develop targeted muscle groups. Another consideration is whether the goal is to increase speed, develop power, improve endurance, produce strength or alter one's appearance.

The *overload and adaptation* principle states that in order for a body system to become more efficient or stronger, it must be stressed beyond its normal levels. In resistance training, this involves stressing the muscles, tendons and ligaments beyond the normal level. The intensity, frequency, and duration of a workout will depend upon an individual's objectives. Specific principles for designing an exercise program will be discussed in a following section. Generally, intensity should be measured by level of fatigue, frequency should be

Variable	Result following resistance training	Result following endurance training
Performance		
Muscle strength	Increases	No change
Muscle endurance	Increases for high power output	Increases for low power output
Aerobic power	No change or increases slightly	Increases
Maximal rate of force production	Increases	No change or decreases
Vertical jump	Ability increases	Ability unchanged
Anaerobic power	Increases	No change
Sprint speed	Improves	No change or improves slightly
Muscle fibers		
Fiber size	Increases	No change or increases slightly
Capillary density	No change or decreases	Increases
Mitochondrial density	Decreases	Increases
Fast heavy-chain myosin	Increases in amount	No change or decreases in amount
Enzyme activity		
Creative phosphokinase	Increases	Increases
Myokinase	Increases	Increases
Phosphofructokinase	Increases	Variable
Lactate dehydrogenase	No change or variable	Variable
Metabolic energy stores		
Stored ATP	Increases	Increases
Stored creatine phosphate	Increases	Increases
Stored glycogen	Increases	Increases
Stored triglycerides	May increase	Increases
Connective tissue		
Ligament strength	Increases	May increase
Tendon strength	Increases	May increase
Collagen content	Variable	May increase
Bone density	Increases	No change or increases
Body composition		
% body fat	Decreases	Decreases
Fat-free body mass	Increases	No change

From: "General Adaptations to Resistance and Endurance Training Programs" by W. J. Kraemer. In *Essentials of Strength Training and Conditioning* (page 131) by T. R. Baechle (Ed.). Champaign, IL: Human Kinetics Publishers. Reprinted by permission.

three times per week with 24 hours rest between workout sessions, and duration should not be more than 45 minutes per session, including warm-up and cool-down.

The *principle of individual differences* is applicable in resistance training as well as cardiovascular training. The primary factor relating to this principle in resistance training is the genetic make up of the skeletal muscular system. The distribution of muscle fiber types will cause individuals to respond differently to the same training stimulus. History of resistance training, age, gender, and, to a limited degree, protein content of the diet can also cause variation in responses. The *principle of reversibility* is applicable to skeletal muscle as well. *Atrophy*, or a decrease in muscle size, will occur very rapidly as a result of disuse.

Program Design for Muscular Fitness

The following are general guidelines for developing an exercise protocol to increase muscular endurance (Cissik, 1998). *Frequency* refers to how often one should lift, with the recommendation being three nonconsecutive days per week. The term *load* defines the amount of weight lifted. This will vary with each individual, with the recommended amount being a weight that will allow 12 to 15 repetitions with good form. If form is compromised, the load should be decreased. *Repetition* is simply the performance of a movement from start to finish one time, and *set* is the specific number of repetitions performed without resting. Twelve to fifteen repetitions per set are recommended while performing two to three sets of each

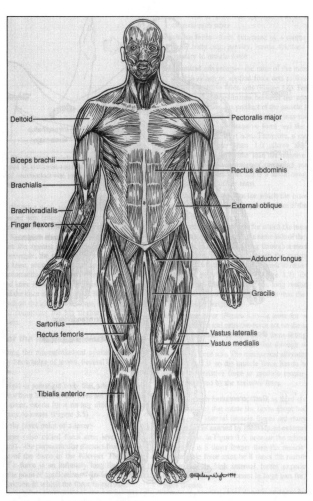

© K. Galasyn-Wright, 1994.

Figure 2.1a Front view of adult male human skeletal musculature

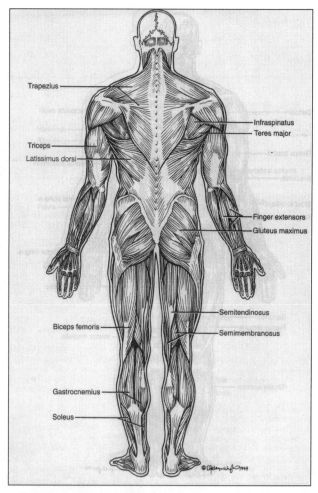

© K. Galasyn-Wright, 1994.

Figure 2.1b Rear view of adult male human skeletal musculature

exercise. *Exercise* is a specific movement designed to work specific muscles or muscle groups. Each exercise session should contain eight to ten different exercises, with at least one being a full body exercise. *Recovery* is the amount of time between each set. Thirty seconds is considered the optimum amount however, taking more time is not detrimental. *Repetition-maximum* is the maximum amount of weight that can be lifted one time without compromising form. *Intensity* is the stress level of the exercise and is expressed as a percent of a one repetition-maximum. The recommended intensity level is less than 70 percent of a one repetition-maximum.

The exercise prescription for developing muscular strength is more intense than for endurance. The number of repetitions decrease from one to eight, with the number of sets increasing from three to five. The percent of the one repetition-maximum that should be lifted increases to 80 to 100 percent. Due to the increase in intensity, the rest period is extended, lasting three to five minutes. Remember the exercise prescription will vary depending on one's goals and objectives for training!

Muscle soreness often accompanies resistance training and will occur at various times during the training process. Muscle soreness that begins late in an exercise session and continues during the immediate recovery period is known as *acute muscle soreness*. This soreness will last only a brief period of time and is typically gone within 24 hours, while *delayed-onset muscle soreness* begins a day or two after the exercise session and can remain for several days. Eccentric contraction seems to be the primary cause of delayed onset muscle soreness. According to Wilmore and Costill (1999), suggested causes of delayed onset muscle soreness include structural damage to muscle cells and inflammatory reactions within the muscles. Muscle soreness can be prevented or minimized by: reducing the eccentric component of muscle action during early training, starting training at a low intensity and gradually increasing it, or beginning with a high-intensity, exhaustive bout, which will cause much soreness initially, but will decrease future pain. During delayed onset muscle soreness, strength production is reduced by as much as fifty percent during the first five days and a reduction in strength can occur for as long as fourteen days. The best technique for prevention of delayed onset

muscle soreness is to maintain an appropriate training program. Diet supplements of vitamin E, an antioxidant, also help to reduce damage to muscle fiber membranes.

As with any type of training program, one should continually monitor one's self for indications of over training. With muscular fitness training, these indicators include a decrease in physical performance, weight loss, increase in muscle soreness, increase in resting heart rate, sleeplessness, nausea after a workout, constant fatigue, and decreased interest in exercise.

Myths and Fallacies Regarding Resistance Training

1. **Myth:** Through resistance training, one will become muscle bound, and flexibility will be lost.
   Fact: Resistance training will increase muscle size, but it does not necessarily make one less flexible. In fact, proper strength training can actually increase flexibility.
2. **Myth:** Resistance training is beneficial in reducing deposits of fat from specific areas on the body, such as in the hips and waist.
   Fact: Fat is not removed from one area of the body by working the muscles in that area. Fat is lost by creating a caloric deficit, through diet, exercise, or a combination of both. The location of fat deposits is determined genetically.
3. **Myth:** Fat will be converted to muscle with resistance training.
   Fact: Fat is not converted to muscle with exercise, nor is muscle converted to fat through disuse. The amount of each can be increased or decreased with resistance training.
4. **Myth:** Dietary supplements will make one bigger and stronger.
   Fact: A balanced diet and the proper resistance training program will increase muscle size and strength. Dietary supplements will only cause the seller's wallet to become bigger.
5. **Myth:** Performance-enhancing drugs such as steroids, growth hormones, and diuretics will help make one fit.

Fact: These drugs are extremely dangerous and potentially fatal! They can contribute to aesthetic changes, but have negative impacts on health and no impact on fitness.

6. **Myth:** Women will become masculine in appearance by participating in resistance training activities.

Fact: Masculinity and femininity are determined through hormones, not through resistance training. Resistance training will cause an increase in muscle tone, which is perceived to increase the attractiveness of both males and females.

Flexibility

A discussion of health-related fitness is incomplete without an explanation of the importance of flexibility. *Flexibility* is defined as the range of motion in any particular joint. Flexibility is also specific to individual joints. For instance, an individual may have complete range of motion in the wrist, but be very limited or stiff in the shoulder. An individual could be very flexible on the right side of the body, and inflexible on the left side. Flexibility exercises should be included in all exercise programs regardless of the objectives. The benefits of maintaining flexibility include having the ability to perform daily activities without developing muscle strains or tears and being able to perform sport skills with enhanced performance. The athlete, whether serious about competition or a weekend recreator, will have a greater ability to perform particular sports skills with an increased range of motion. Flexibility also helps to prevent injuries through a reduction in strains and muscle tears. It is especially important to include flexibility exercises in a muscular fitness workout! The increase in muscle strength and size will contribute to a decrease in flexibility unless measures are taken to counter that affect. Several factors can have an impact on the amount of flexibility an individual can achieve, including gender, age, genetic composition, and previous or current injury.

Stretching exercises are identified through three specific categories. *Ballistic stretching* involves dynamic movements, or what is commonly referred to as "bouncing." Ballistic stretching is not recommended as a means to improve flexibility. This type of stretch actually stimulates receptors in the muscle which are designed to help prevent injury due to over extending the muscle. Thus, the ballistic stretch actually causes the muscle to contract rather than relax, and often contributes to muscle soreness. A more appropriate type of muscular stretching is identified as *static stretching*. Static stretching involves slowly moving the joint to the point of mild uncomfortableness in the muscle and maintaining that angle for 30 seconds before allowing the muscle to relax. The entire procedure should be repeated several times for maximum benefit. A third type of stretching activity is called *proprioceptive neuromuscular facilitation*. This activity requires a partner to provide resistance. The basic formula for this activity is to isometrically resist against a partner using the muscle groups surrounding a particular joint, causing contraction, and then relaxing the same muscle group. For example, in stretching the hamstring, both the hamstrings and the quadriceps will be contracted, and then relaxed. This contraction and relaxation process will increase the range of motion in the hamstrings.

Basic principles to remember regarding flexibility:

1. it is specific to each joint; therefore, stretching activities must be identified and practiced for each joint;

2. maintaining an adequate amount of flexibility will decrease the likelihood of injuries;

3. flexibility increases when the muscle temperature is elevated and decreases when the muscle is cold; and

4. experiencing pain in a muscle while performing flexibility exercises is not necessary and could potentially be a warning sign of inappropriate stretching technique.

References

Cissik, J.M. 1998. *The Basics of Strength Training*. New York: McGraw-Hill Companies, Inc.

Corbin, C. B., and Lindsey, R. 1994. *Concepts of Fitness and Wellness with Laboratories*. Madison, WI: Brown & Benchmark.

Floyd, P.A., Mimms, S.E. and Yelding-Howard, C. 1998. *Personal Health Perspectives and Lifestyles*. Englewood, Colorado: Morton Publishing Company.

Fox, E., Bowers, R., and Merle, F. 1989. *The Physiological Basis for Exercise and Sport.* 5th ed. Madison, WI: WCB Brown & Benchmark Publishers.

Kimbrough, S. K. 1997. *Fitness & Conditioning.* Stipes Publishing L.L.C.

McArdle, W.D., Katch, F.I. and Katch, V.L. 1999. *Exercise Physiology Energy, Nutrition, and Human Performance.* Baltimore, MD.: Williams and Wilkins.

Pate, R., Pratt, M., Blair, S., Haskell, W., Macera, C., Bouchard, C., Buchner, D., Ettinger, W., Heath, G., King, A., Driska, A., Leon, A., Marcus, B., Morris, J., Paffenbarger, R., Patrick, K., Pollock, M., Rippe, J., Sallis, J., and Wilmore, J. 1995. Physical Activity and Public Health: A Recommendation from the Centers for Disease Control and Prevention and the American College of Sports Medicine. *Journal of the American Medical Association*, 273: 402–407.

Physical Activity and Health: A Report of the Surgeon General. 1996. Atlanta: U.S. Department of Health and Human Services, Centers for Disease Control and Prevention, National Center for Chronic Disease Prevention and Health Promotion.

Pollock, M.L., Gaesser, G.A., Butcher, J.D., Despres, J-P., Dishman, R.K., Franklin, B.A., and Garber, C.E. 1998. ACSM Position Stand on the Recommended Quantity and Quality of Exercise for Developing and Maintaining Cardiorespiratory and Muscular Fitness, and Flexibility in Adults. *Medicine & Science in Sports & Exercise*, 30: 975–991.

Sharkey, Brian J. 1997. *Fitness and Health.* Champaign, IL: Human Kinetics Publishing.

Sieg, K.W., and Adams, S.P. (1985). *Illustrated Essentials of Musculoskeletal Anatomy.* Gainesville, FL: Megabooks Inc.

Wilmore, Jack H. and Costill, David L. 1999. *Physiology of Sport and Exercise.* Champaign, IL: Human Kinetics Publishing Company.

Contacts

American College of Sports Medicine (ACSM)
http://www.acsm.org/sportsmed

American Running and Fitness Association
http://www.arfa.org

American Heart Association
www.americanheart.org/statistics/

American Medical Association
http://www.ama-assn.org

Centers for Disease Control and Prevention
http://www.cdc.gov/nccdphp/sgr/mm.thm

Fitness World
http://www.fitnessworld.com

National Institute of Arthritis and Musculoskeletal and Skin Diseases
http://www.healthfinder.gov/text/orgs/hr0036.htm

President's Council on Physical Fitness and Sports
Fitness Fundamentals
http://www.hoptechno.com/book11.htm

President's Council on Physical Fitness and Sports
The Link Between Physical Activity and Morbidity and Mortality
http://www.cdc.gov/nccdphp/sgr/mm.htm

President's Council on Physical Fitness and Sports
Tucker Center—Women in Sport
http://www.kls.coled.umn.edu/crgws/

Results from the President's Council on Physical Fitness
http://www.girsite.org/Html/nike2.htm

Shape Up America!
http://www.shapeup.org

Notebook Activities

PAR-Q and YOU

Calculating Your Activity Index

Determine an Accurate Heart Rate

Developing an Exercise Program for Cardiorespiratory Endurance

Assessing Your Current Level of Muscular Endurance

Assessing Your Current Level of Muscular Strength

■ Safety of Exercise Participation: PAR-Q
PAR-Q & You
(A Questionnaire for People Aged 15 to 69)

Regular physical activity is fun and healthy, and increasingly more people are starting to become more active every day. Being more active is very safe for most people. However, some people should check with their doctor before they start becoming much more physically active.

If you are planning to become much more physically active than you are now, start by answering the seven questions in the box below. If you are between the ages of 15 and 69, the PAR-Q will tell you if you should check with your doctor before you start. If you are over 69 years of age, and you are not used to being very active, check with your doctor.

Common sense is your best guide when you answer these questions. Please read the questions carefully and answer each one honestly: check YES or NO.

YES	NO	
☐	☐	1. Has your doctor ever said that you have a heart condition *and* that you should only do physical activity recommended by a doctor?
☐	☐	2. Do you feel pain in your chest when you do physical activity?
☐	☐	3. In the past month, have you had chest pain when you were not doing physical activity?
☐	☐	4. Do you lose your balance because of dizziness or do you ever lose consciousness?
☐	☐	5. Do you have a bone or joint problem that could be made worse by a change in your physical activity?
☐	☐	6. Is your doctor currently prescribing drugs (for example, water pills) for your blood pressure or heart condition?
☐	☐	7. Do you know of *any other reason* why you should not do physical activity?

If

you

answered

YES to one or more questions

Talk with your doctor by phone or in person BEFORE you start becoming much more physically active or BEFORE you have a fitness appraisal. Tell your doctor about the PAR-Q and which questions you answered YES.

- You may be able to do any activity you want—as long as you start slowly and build up gradually. Or, you may need to restrict your activities to those which are safe for you. Talk with your doctor about the kinds of activities you wish to participate in and follow his/her advice.
- Find out which community programs are safe and helpful for you.

NO to all questions

If you answered NO honestly to *all* PAR-Q questions, you can be reasonably sure that you can:
- start becoming much more physically active—begin slowly and build up gradually. This is the safest and easiest way to go.
- take part in a fitness appraisal—this is an excellent way to determine your basic fitness so that you can plan the best way for you to live actively.

DELAY BECOMING MUCH MORE ACTIVE:
- if you are not feeling well because of a temporary illness such as a cold or a fever—wait until you feel better, or
- if you are or may be pregnant—talk to your doctor before you start becoming more active.

Please note: If your health changes so that you then answer YES to any of the above questions, tell your fitness or health professional. Ask whether you should change your physical activity plan.

Informed Use of the PAR-Q: The Canadian Society for Exercise Physiology, Health Canada, and their agents assume no liability for persons who undertake physical activity, and if in doubt after completing this questionnaire, consult your doctor prior to physical activity.

You are encouraged to copy the PAR-Q but only if you use the entire form.

Note: If the PAR-Q is being given to a person before he or she participates in a physical activity program or a fitness appraisal, this section may be used for legal or administrative purposes.

I have read, understood and completed this questionnaire. Any questions I had were answered to my full satisfaction.

NAME _____

SIGNATURE _____ DATE _____

SIGNATURE OF PARENT _____ WITNESS _____

or GUARDIAN (for participants under the age of majority)

Supported by: Health   Santé
Canada   Canada

■ Calculating your Activity Index

Frequency: How often do you exercise?

If you exercise:	Your frequency score is:
Less than 1 time a week	0
1 time a week	1
2 times a week	2
3 times a week	3
4 times a week	4
5 or more times a week	5

Duration: How long do you exercise?

If your total duration of exercise is:	Your duration score is:
Less than 5 minutes	0
5–14 minutes	1
15–29 minutes	2
30–44 minutes	3
45–59 minutes	4
60 minutes or more	5

Intensity: How hard do you exercise?

If exercise results in:	Your intensity score is:
No change in pulse from resting level	0
Slight increase in pulse from resting level	1
Slight increase in pulse and breathing	2
Moderate increase in pulse and breathing	3
Intermittent heavy breathing and sweating	4
Sustained heavy breathing and sweating	5

Multiply your three scores:

Frequency _____ × Duration _____ × Intensity _____ = Activity index _____

To determinue your activity index, refer to the following table:

If your activity index is:	Your estimated level of activity is:
Less than 15	Sedentary
15–24	Low active
25–40	Moderate active
41–60	Active
Over 60	High active

■ Determining an Accurate Heart Rate

Procedure: Using the first two fingers on either hand, press gently on the radial artery (wrist, thumb side) until you can feel a consistent pulse. Press gently on the carotid artery (side of the neck) until you can feel a consistent pulse. Identify a partner and complete the chart below.

Radial Pulse (self)

_____ 15 seconds × 4 = _____ bpm

_____ 30 seconds × 2 = _____ bpm

_____ 60 seconds × 1 = _____ bpm

Radial Pulse (partner)

_____ 15 seconds × 4 = _____ bpm

_____ 30 seconds × 2 = _____ bpm

_____ 60 seconds × 1 = _____ bpm

Carotid Pulse (self)

_____ 15 seconds × 4 = _____ bpm

_____ 30 seconds × 2 = _____ bpm

_____ 60 seconds × 1 = _____ bpm

Carotid Pulse (partner)

_____ 15 seconds × 4 = _____ bpm

_____ 30 seconds × 2 = _____ bpm

_____ 60 seconds × 1 = _____ bpm

■ Developing an Exercise Program for Cardiorespiratory Endurance

Please print:

Goals: Identify three goals you want to accomplish as a result of this program. Goals should be accomplished by the end of the semester.

1. _____
   _____

2. _____
   _____

3. _____
   _____

Activities: Identify three different activities you will perform.

1. _____
2. _____
3. _____

Duration: Fill in an amount of time for each exercise session and activity.

Activity   Duration

1. _____   _____
2. _____   _____
3. _____   _____

Intensity: Complete the blanks below.

Maximum heart rate: 220 – _____ = _____ bpm
                              age

55% intensity = _____ bpm × 0.55 = _____ bpm
                    (MHR)

90% intensity = _____ bpm × 0.90 = _____ bpm
                    (MHR)

Target heart rate range = _____ bpm to _____ bpm
                              55% bpm   90% bpm

Frequency: How many days each week will you exercise? _____

Recording: Complete the following form for four consecutive weeks.

Exercise Record

Date	Activity	Duration in Minutes	Heart Rate bpm last minute	Intensity exercise HR ÷ MHR

■ Assessing Your Current Level of Muscular Endurance

Push-up Test:

Men should use the standard push up position with hands shoulder width apart and feet on the floor. Women may modify the standard push up position by putting their knees on the floor. Complete as many push ups as possible without stopping and evaluate your performance according to the following.

MEN					WOMEN				
Age	20s	30s	40s	50s	Age	20s	30s	40s	50s
Good	40	36	30	27	Good	38	33	27	22
Fair	35	30	25	22	Fair	32	27	22	18
Poor	30	25	21	18	Poor	27	22	18	15

Curl-up Test:

Begin by lying on your back, arms by your sides with palms down and on the floor and fingers straight. Your knees should be bent at about 90 degrees, with your feet 12 inches away from your buttocks. To perform a curl up, curl your head and upper back upward keeping your arms straight. Slide your fingers forward along the floor until you touch the back of your heels. Then curl back down until your back and head reach the floor. Palms, feet and buttocks remain on the floor the entire time. Perform as many curl ups as you can in one minute without stopping to rest and evaluate your performance according to the following.

MEN					WOMEN				
Age	20s	30s	40s	50s	Age	20s	30s	40s	50s
Good	25	25	25	25	Good	25	25	25	25
Fair	22	22	21	19	Fair	22	21	20	15
Poor	13	13	11	09	Poor	13	11	06	04

■ Assessing Your Current Level of Muscular Strength

Bench Press Test:

Do not use free weights for this test. On a weight machine set the machine for a weight that is slightly lower than the amount you believe you can lift one time. Adjust the weight either up or down until you determine the amount of weight you can lift one time. You will need to rest between each attempt. Once you have identified your maximum bench press weight, divide the number by your body weight and use the following chart to determine your upper body muscular strength.

MEN				
Age	20s	30s	40s	50s
Good	≥ 1.6	≥ 1.3	≥ 1.1	≥ 1.0
Fair	1.3	1.1	0.6	0.8
Poor	≤ 0.8	≤ 0.7	≤ 0.7	≤ 0.6

WOMEN				
Age	20s	30s	40s	50s
Good	≥ 1.0	≥ 0.8	≥ 0.7	≥ 0.6
Fair	0.7	0.6	0.6	0.5
Poor	≤ 0.5	≤ 0.4	≤ 0.4	≤ 0.3

Leg Press Test:

On a leg press machine set the machine following the same procedures as you used for the bench press test. Once you determine your maximum leg press weight, divide the number by your body weight and use the following chart to determine your lower body muscular strength.

MEN				
Age	20s	30s	40s	50s
Good	≥ 2.3	≥ 2.1	≥ 2.0	≥ 1.8
Fair	2.1	1.9	1.8	1.7
Poor	≤ 1.6	≤ 1.5	≤ 1.4	≤ 1.3

WOMEN				
Age	20s	30s	40s	50s
Good	≥ 1.9	≥ 1.6	≥ 1.5	≥ 1.4
Fair	1.67	1.46	1.36	1.24
Poor	≤ 1.2	≤ 1.0	≤ 0.9	≤ 0.8

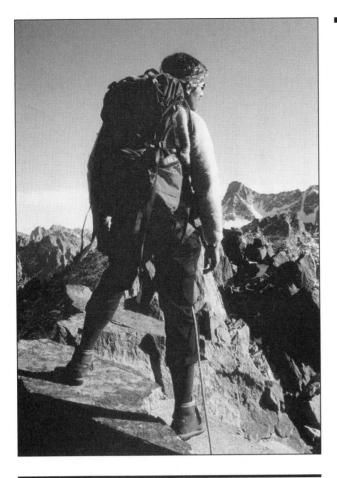

Chapter Three

Hypokinetic Conditions

"The sovereign invigorator of the body is exercise, and of all the exercises walking is the best."

—Thomas Jefferson

OBJECTIVES

Students will be able to:

- identify five major diseases associated with cardiovascular disease

- identify the major hypokinetic diseases afflicting Americans

- identify ways to prevent hypokinetic conditions

- define obesity

- identify three ways to prevent becoming obese

- identify three ways to prevent low back pain

The term hypokinetic was first coined by Kraus and Rabb in 1961. Hypokinetic literally means too little activity. In the past infectious diseases such as polio, small pox and tuberculosis were a large-scale threat to survival. Now the leading causes of death are diseases that are associated with too little activity. Western culture has promoted a lifestyle of limited physical activity. Simply changing an individual's lifestyle to one that includes more physical activity can reduce the incidence of many disease processes. Regular activity can decrease the potential of developing a hypokinetic disease. For example,

- Expending 500–1,000 calories exercising each week can decrease overall health risk by 22%.

- Expending 1,000–2,000 calories exercising each week can decrease overall health risk more and increase cardiovascular fitness levels moderately.

- Expending 2,000–3,500 calories exercising each week can decrease overall health risk by 38–54% and increase cardiovascular fitness levels significantly over a period of time.

• Expending beyond 3,500 calories exercising each week can cause a higher risk of musculoskeletal injuries and burnout (Corbin and Lindsey, 1997).

The Center for Disease Control (CDC) reports that lifestyle is the single greatest factor affecting longevity of life. America's children are more sedentary and at higher risk for developing hypokinetic diseases than their parents or grandparents. This is partially due to technology and the ease at which tasks are performed. For example, many individuals no longer need to make a full day trip to the library and carry books around for days in order to complete an assignment, cash machines enable people to get money without getting out of their car, and cable TV and remote controls allow for hours of mental entertainment without expending any extra calories.

Documentation supports the benefits of a healthier lifestyle.

The *American Heart Association* (AHA) identified inactivity as a major risk factor in 1992. Only after much thought, reflection and research did the AHA change risk factors to add inactivity.

Healthy People 2000—(National Health Promotion and Disease Prevention Objectives) Developed statements by expert groups representing over 300 national organizations that include realistic health goals to be achieved by the year 2000.

Surgeon General's Report (1996) traced the link between physical activity and good health. This document suggests that a healthy lifestyle is the most critical element for optimal wellness.

Centers for Disease Control provides scientific and technical leadership and assistance to help states, national organizations and professional groups reduce major risk factors associated with chronic diseases in the U.S.

Types of Hypokinetic Conditions

Cardiovascular Disease (CVD)

The cardiovascular system is responsible for delivering oxygen and other nutrients to the body. The major components of the cardiovascular system are the heart, blood and the vessels that carry the

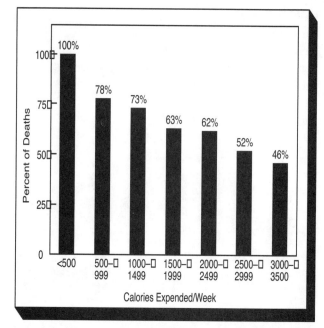

Data from C. Bouchard et al, *Exercise Fitness and Health.* Champaign, IL: Human Kinetics Publishers, 1990.

FIGURE 3.1 Deaths decrease as caloric expenditure increases. The baseline death rate was established for inactive people [<500 calories].

blood. Cardiovascular disease is a "catch-all" phrase that includes several disease processes. First, the heart muscle may become damaged or lose its ability to contract effectively. Also the vessels which supply the heart with oxygen may become blocked or damaged and subsequently compromise the heart muscle. Finally, the peripheral vascular system (all of the vessels outside the heart) may become damaged and decrease the heart's ability to provide oxygen to other parts of the body. There are many factors which can affect a person's risk for developing cardiovascular disease. Variables such as age, gender, race, and genetic makeup may place one at a higher or lower risk and cannot be changed. These can be termed unalterable risk factors. However, there are many other risk factors that can be altered. These include but are not limited to: diet, drug use, smoking history, cholesterol levels, obesity, high blood pressure, and last but definitely not least, physical inactivity. The Surgeon General's report (1996) placed physical inactivity as a significant risk factor for cardiovascular diseases and other health disorders. This is a critical point, since activity level is a risk factor that can be easily modified and is often overlooked. Increasing an individual's activity level can prevent many of the diseases discussed in this chapter. Cardiovascular disease is the leading cause of death in the United States. In 1995 approximately 42% of the deaths in the U.S. were from some type of cardiovascular disease. Every 34 seconds someone dies of a cardiovascular disease (American Heart Association, 1995).

Consistent physical activity affects cardiovascular disease by one or more of the following mechanisms:

- Improved cardiovascular fitness and health
- Greater lean (fat-free) body mass
- Improved strength and muscular endurance
- Stronger heart muscle
- Lower heart rate
- Increased oxygen to the brain
- Reduced blood fat including LDLs
- Increased protective HDLs
- Delayed development of atherosclerosis
- Increased work capacity
- Improved peripheral circulation
- Improved coronary circulation
- Reduced risk of heart attack
- Reduced risk of stroke
- Reduced risk of hypertension
- Greater chance of surviving a heart attack
- Greater oxygen carrying capacity of the blood

Arteriosclerosis

Arteriosclerosis is a term used to describe the hardening of the arteries. Healthy arteries are elastic and will dilate and constrict with changes in blood flow due to demands with exercise or rest. This allows for proper maintenance of blood pressure. Hardened, non-elastic arteries do not expand with blood flow and can increase intrarterial pressure causing high blood pressure. Both high blood pressure and arteriosclerosis increase the risk of an aneurysm. With an aneurysm, the artery loses its integrity and balloons out under the pressure created by the pumping heart, in much the same way as an old garden hose might if placed under pressure. If an aneurysm occurs in the vessels of the brain a stroke might occur. Aneurysms in the large vessels can place a person at risk of sudden death.

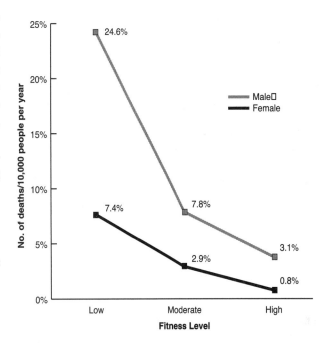

Data source: Blair et al, Physical fitness and all-cause mortality: A prospective study of healthy men and women. *Journal of the American Medical Association* 262(17): 2395–2401, 1989.

FIGURE 3.2 Relationship between different levels of fitness and death due to cardiovascular disease among men and women.
(Adapted from S. N. Blair, H. W. Kohl III, R. S. Paffenbarger, Jr., D. G. C.ark, K. H. Cooper, and L. W. Gibbons. Physical fitness and all-cause mortality: A prospective study of healthy men and women.)

Obviously, maintaining normal elasticity of the arteries is very important.

Atherosclerosis

Atherosclerosis is the long-term build up of fatty deposits and other substances such as cholesterol, cellular waste products, calcium and fibrin (clotting material in the blood) on the interior walls of arteries. (See Figure 3.3) These eventually form plaque deposits and are responsible for 85% of all cardiovascular deaths (Bishop, 1999). The leading theory states that plaque develops when the endothelium is damaged due to major fluctuations in blood pressure, increased levels of blood triglycerides and cholesterol as well as cigarette smoking. These conditions accelerate the development of atherosclerosis, which can start at a very young age. Due to this plaque development, the flow of blood

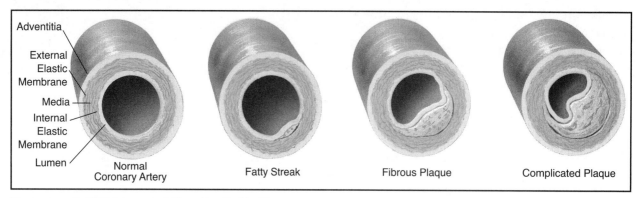

Illustrations © 1997 Anatomical Chart Co., Skokie, IL

FIGURE 3.3 Atherosclerosis is an accumulation of plaque deposits in the lining of the arteries. This sequence of drawings illustrates a gradual build-up of atherosclerotic plaque, which, in the long term, reduces circulation of blood. This increases the risk of heart attack, stroke, and other serious arterial diseases.

within the artery decreases because the diameter of the vessel is lessened. This may create a partial or total blockage (called an occlusion) which may cause high blood pressure, a heart attack or stroke. This process can occur in any vessel of the body. If it occurs outside of the brain or heart, it is termed peripheral vascular disease.

Peripheral Vascular Disease

Peripheral Vascular Disease is simply a term attributed to disease of the peripheral vessels. The lack of proper circulation may cause fluids to pool in the extremities. Associated leg pain, cramping, numbness, tingling, coldness, and loss of hair to affected limbs are common signs. The restrictions in blood flow are typically caused by years of arteriosclerosis and atherosclerosis in the vessels of the extremities. The risk factors are the same as those for cardiovascular disease. One difference is that the disease process may progress extensively before the affected person begins to notice any problems. The heart and brain are much more sensitive to compromised blood flow than the extremities.

Hypertension

Hypertension is high blood pressure, which affects about 50 million Americans (American Heart Association, 1998). Hypertension has been called the "silent killer" since it can progress without any symptoms. A "textbook normal" adult's blood pressure is 120/80. The top number is the systolic read-

ing, which represents the pressure when the heart is contracting and forcing the blood through the arteries. The bottom number or diastolic reading is the force of the blood on the arteries while the heart is relaxing between beats. Normal values can deviate from the 120/80 reading significantly. However, values above 140/90 indicate a higher risk. Often hypertension cannot be cured, but can be successfully treated. Most people with hypertension have additional risk factors for cardiovascular disease. Some of the risk factors for high blood pressure include Hispanic or African American cultures, older age, family history, a diet high in fat and salt, stress, obesity and lack of exercise.

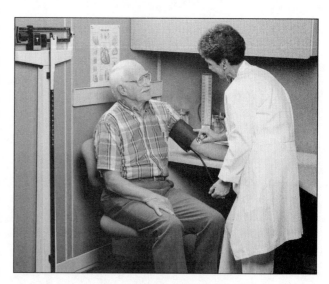

TABLE 3.1. Standards for Classification of Blood Pressure for Adults age 18 Years and Older

Category	Systolic (mm Hg)	Diastolic (mm Hg)
Normal	< 130	< 85
High Normal	130–139	85–89
Hypertension		
Stage 1 (Mild)	140–159	90–99
Stage 2 (Moderate)	160–179	100–109
Stage 3 (Severe)	180–209	110–119
Stage 4 (Very Severe)	> 210	> 120

Source: National Institutes of Health, *The Fifth Report of the Joint National Committee on Detection, Evaluation and Treatment of High Blood Pressure*, U.S. Dept. of Health and Human Services: NIH Publication No. 93-1088, January, 1993.

Heart Attack

A heart attack or myocardial infarction occurs when an artery that provides the heart muscle with oxygen becomes blocked or flow is decreased. The area of the heart muscle served by that artery does not receive adequate oxygen and becomes injured and may eventually die (See Figure 3.4). The heart attack may be so small as to be imperceptible by the victim, or so massive that the victim will die. Women who smoke and take oral contraceptives are 10 times more likely to have a heart attack (Payne, 1995). Some findings suggest that coronary collateral circulation is increased with regular physical activity (Corbin, 1997). This may decrease the risk of having a heart attack as well as increase the chances of survival if a heart attack does occur, because the new vessels, which form as a result of

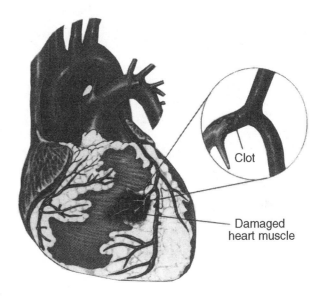

American Academy of Orthopaedic Surgeons, *Emergency Care and Transportation of the Sick and Injured*, Seventh Edition, Sudbury, MA: Jones and Bartlett Publishers. www.jbpub.com. Reprinted with permission.

FIGURE 3.4 An acute myocardial infarction occurs when a blood clot prevents blood flow to an area of the heart muscle. If left untreated this can result in death of heart tissue.

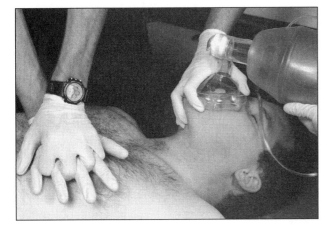

exercise, can take over if a major coronary artery is blocked. Since 1951, the death rate from heart attacks has declined by 51%, yet more Americans die from coronary artery disease than from any other disease.

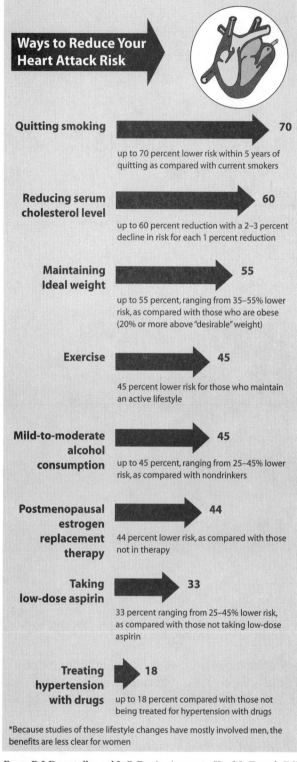

Ways to Reduce Your Heart Attack Risk

Quitting smoking — 70
up to 70 percent lower risk within 5 years of quitting as compared with current smokers

Reducing serum cholesterol level — 60
up to 60 percent reduction with a 2–3 percent decline in risk for each 1 percent reduction

Maintaining Ideal weight — 55
up to 55 percent, ranging from 35–55% lower risk, as compared with those who are obese (20% or more above "desirable" weight)

Exercise — 45
45 percent lower risk for those who maintain an active lifestyle

Mild-to-moderate alcohol consumption — 45
up to 45 percent, ranging from 25–45% lower risk, as compared with nondrinkers

Postmenopausal estrogen replacement therapy — 44
44 percent lower risk, as compared with those not in therapy

Taking low-dose aspirin — 33
33 percent ranging from 25–45% lower risk, as compared with those not taking low-dose aspirin

Treating hypertension with drugs — 18
up to 18 percent compared with those not being treated for hypertension with drugs

*Because studies of these lifestyle changes have mostly involved men, the benefits are less clear for women

From R.J. Donatelle and L.G. Davis, *Access to Health*, Fourth Edition. Copyright © 1996. All rights reserved. Reprinted by permission of Allyn and Bacon.

FIGURE 3.5 Estimated Average Reduction in Risk for Heart Attack*
*Estimated risk reductions refer to the independent contribution of each risk factor to heart attack and do not address the wide range of known or hypothesized reactions among them.

Stroke

Stroke, or more recently called "brain attack" is the third leading cause of death (Rosato, 1994). This occurs when the vessels that supply the brain with nutrients become damaged or occluded and the brain tissue dies (See Figure 3.6). Like heart disease, strokes may take years to develop. Stroke has the same risk factors as heart disease. Like heart disease, conditions favorable to stroke also respond favorably to exercise. Ischemic (thrombosis and embolism) strokes are the most common form of stroke (75–85%) and occur as a result of a blockage to the cerebral artery (Hafen, Karren and Frandsen, 1999). The process is similar to that which occurs in a heart attack. The second most common type of stroke is a cerebral hemorrhage or aneurysm, in which the vessel may rupture and cause bleeding inside the head and result in pressure on the brain. Fifteen to twenty-five percent of strokes are caused by hemorrhage. The least common form of stroke results from compression which can occur as a result of a hemorrhage or brain tumor. African Americans have a 60% greater risk of a stroke than Caucasians (Corbin, 1997).

Risk Factors For Cardiovascular Disease

Cigarette Smoking—Smokers have five times the risk of developing cardiovascular disease than do nonsmokers (Corbin, 1997). Cigarette smoking is the most "potent" of the preventable risk factors. Smoking accounts for 1/2 of the female deaths due to heart attack before the age of 55 (Rosato, 1994).

Hypertension—The American Heart Association (1998) reports that approximately 50 Million American adults and children have high blood pressure. Reports from the Harvard Alumni Study (1986) show that subjects who did not engage in vigorous sports or activity were 35% more likely to develop hypertension than those who were regularly active.

Cholesterol—Dietary cholesterol contributes to blood serum cholesterol (cholesterol circulating in the blood) which can contribute to heart disease. Every one percent reduction in serum cholesterol can result in a 2 to 3 % reduction in the risk of heart disease (Rosato, 1994). To lower cholesterol, reduce intake of dietary saturated fat, increase consumption of soluble fiber, maintain a

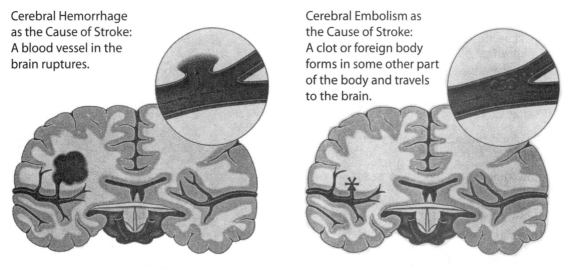

Cerebral Hemorrhage as the Cause of Stroke: A blood vessel in the brain ruptures.

Cerebral Embolism as the Cause of Stroke: A clot or foreign body forms in some other part of the body and travels to the brain.

STROKE

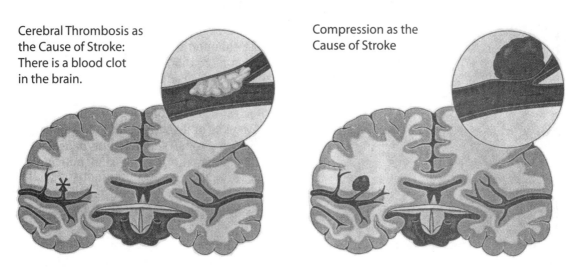

Cerebral Thrombosis as the Cause of Stroke: There is a blood clot in the brain.

Compression as the Cause of Stroke

From B.O. Hafen, K.J. Karren and K.J. Frandsen, *First Aid for Colleges and Universities*, Seventh Edition. Copyright © 1999. All rights reserved. Reprinted by permission of Allyn and Bacon.

FIGURE 3.6 Causes of stroke

healthy weight, do not smoke and exercise regularly.

Inactivity—Physical inactivity can be very debilitating to the human body. The changes brought about by the aging process can be simulated in a few weeks of bed rest for a young person. Aerobic exercise on a regular basis can favorably influence the other modifiable risk factors for heart disease. Consistent, moderate amounts of physical activity can promote health and longevity. The Surgeon General's report states that as little as 150 extra calories expended daily exercising can dramatically decrease CVD risk.

Other Contributing Risk Factors

Obesity is highly correlated to heart disease. Mild to moderate obesity is associated with an increase in risk of CVD (Rosato, 1994). Fat distribution can also predict higher risk. A waist to hip ratio that is greater than 1.0 for men and greater than 0.8 for women constitutes a higher risk because abdominal fat is more easily mobilized and dispersed into the bloodstream, thereby elevating serum cholesterol levels.

Diabetes—More than 80% of diabetics die of some form of CVD (Rosato, 1994). Exercise is critical to help increase the sensitivity of the body's cells to insulin.

Stress—Although difficult to measure in concrete form, is considered a factor in the development and acceleration of CVD. Without stress management techniques, constant stress can manifest itself in a physical nature in the human body. Stress contributes to many of today's illnesses.

Triglycerides—Most of the fat in the human body is stored in the form of triglycerides. Elevated triglyceride levels are thought to increase CVD risk by being involved in the plaque formation of atherosclerosis.

Uncontrollable Risk Factors

Age—Risk of CVD rises as a person ages.

Gender—Men have a higher risk than women do until women reach post-menopausal age. Remember that CVD is an equal opportunity killer!

Heredity—A family history of heart disease will increase risk.

Obesity

Obesity is defined as a weight 20% or more over ideal body weight and is often accompanied by a loss of functional ability.

- Body fat measuring >25% for men and >32% for women is considered obese (Bishop, 1999).
- Obesity is primarily caused by a hypokinetic condition. Obesity causes, contributes to and complicates many of the diseases which afflict Americans.

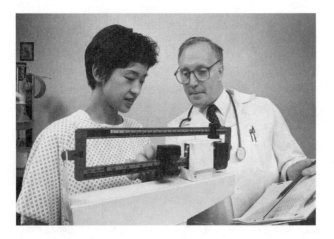

- Obesity is associated with a shortened life, serious organ impairment, awkward movements, poor relationships and a higher risk of cardiovascular disease, diabetes, as well as colon and breast cancer.
- Twice as many children were overweight in the 1990s as in the 1960s (Corbin, 1997).
- There is only a two to three percent success rate for people who lose weight to actually maintain the weight loss (Texas A&M University Human Nutrition Conference, 1998). The key is to exercise, maintain a healthy diet throughout your life and avoid gaining excess weight.
- Exercise greatly increases the likelihood of success with a maintenance program after weight loss.
- Creeping obesity is a gradual increase of fat content as activity decreases with age. This typically results in a ½ to 1 lb. of fat gain per year.

Activity is the optimal way to manage current weight or successfully lose weight.

Causes of Obesity

- Caloric intake exceeds caloric expenditure, which is either overeating, lack of activity or both.
- Genetically we are predisposed to a certain somatotype, fat distribution, size and weight. An individual's behavior can help to modify these characteristics.
- Glandular disorders affect two percent of the obese population which can be treated medically (Corbin, 1997).
- Thyroid disease is one that can slow a person's metabolic rate.

Childhood Obesity Is a Concern

- Infants can be overfed, toddlers can be pacified with candy and teenagers love soft drinks and junk food.
- Overweight parents are more likely to have overweight children as they learn eating and activity patterns from parents.
- Nineteen out of twenty overweight teenagers are overweight adults (Texas A&M University Human Nutrition Conference, 1998).

- Twenty-one percent of U.S. teenagers today are overweight, which is an increase of six percent from the 1970s (Donatelle, 1996).

- Automation in the society helps us all "save calories" both at work and school, as well as at home. Labor saving devices are a convenience but also a mechanism for people to save energy, therefore calories.

- Weight gain occurs with inactivity; activity is the best way to reduce the size of fat stores.

- Most people who lose weight by dieting alone regain their lost pounds, and often additional pounds as well. This is called "yo-yo" dieting which results in a rebound effect and is stressful to the heart. Yo-yo dieting often makes it even harder to lose the weight the next time because the percentage of body fat creeps up each time weight is regained.

Physiological Response to Obesity

- More blood vessels are needed to circulate blood.

- The heart has to pump harder, therefore increasing blood pressure.

- Extra weight can be tough on the musculoskeletal joints, causing problems with arthritis, gout, bone and joint diseases, varicose veins, gallbladder disease, as well as complications during pregnancy.

- Obesity increases most cancer risks (Bishop, 1999).

Cancer

- Data exists linking inactivity with a higher risk of rectal cancer (Rosato, 1994).

- Inactive individuals have a 50–250% greater chance of developing colon cancer than active people (Corbin, 1997).

- Fit individuals may have a decreased risk of reproductive organ cancers (Bishop, 1999).

- Many health professionals agree that approximately 80% of all cancers could be avoided by healthy lifestyle choices (Rosato, 1994).

- Thirty-five percent of the total cancer death toll is associated with diet (Rosato, 1994).

- Activity helps those with cancer lead more fulfilling and productive lives.

"Exercise is a known remedy for the weakness and low spirits that cancer patients experience during their recovery. It boosts energy and endurance, and also builds confidence and optimism. But, within the past five years, several medical investigations have revealed a surprising new fact: Exercise may also help prevent cancer"

(Rosato, 1994).

"Recognition of the potential of exercise to prevent cancer came in 1985 when the American Cancer Society began recommending exercise to protect against cancer"

(Rosato, 1994).

Diabetes

Diabetes is the sixth leading cause of death in people over 40 (Corbin, 1997). Exercise plays an important role in managing this disease, as exercise helps control body fat and improves insulin sensitivity and glucose tolerance. The mortality rate is greater in diabetics with CVD—males are two to three times more likely to die and females are three to seven times more likely to die than their non-diabetic counterparts (Rosato, 1994). Eighty percent of the adults who develop diabetes are obese (Rosato, 1994).

Low Back Pain

More than eight out of ten Americans will suffer some back-related pain at some point in their lifetime (Corbin, 1997). Low back pain is epidemic throughout the world and is the major cause of disability in people aged 20-45 in the United States (Donatelle, et al., 1996). Ninety percent of back injuries occur in the lumbar region (Donatelle, et al., 1996).

Facts About Back Pain

- Backache is the second leading medical complaint when visiting a physician (Corbin, 1997).

- The National Safety Council data indicates that the back is the most frequently injured of all the body parts, with the injury rate double that of other body parts.

- Thirty to seventy percent of all Americans have recurring back problems; two million Americans cannot hold a job as a result (Corbin, 1997).
- Back pain is the most frequent cause of inactivity in individuals under the age of 45 (Corbin, 1997).
- Intervertebral disks can suffer degeneration from overuse, which is more common in men than women.

Common Causes of Back Pain

- Lack of physical fitness.
- Poor posture, balance, strength and flexibility.
- Weak abdominal muscles, tight hip flexors and hamstrings. Be sure to stretch hip flexors and hamstrings daily as well as strengthen abdominals by doing sit-ups at least three times a week.
- Improper lifting, work habits, heredity and disease such as scoliosis.
- Occupational risks—employees new to a job most often injure their back.

Osteoporosis

Osteoporosis is a disease characterized by a loss of bone density which afflicts 24 million Americans annually. One out of two women over 50 will have an osteoporosis-related fracture at some point in her life (http://www.osteo.org/osteo.html). This disease is frequently seen in older Caucasian women. African Americans have bones that are 10% more dense than Caucasians (Greenberg, 1998).

Some Causes of this Disease

- A reduction in calcium intake, either orally or inefficient absorption due to lack of vitamin D or consuming too much caffeine; more than 75% of adults do not consume enough calcium on a daily basis (Bishop, 1999).
- Inactivity results in a loss of muscle tone and the stimulation that is needed to facilitate bone growth.

- Decreased estrogen levels due to menopause.

Current Recommendations

- 1200 mg of calcium/day
- Engage in daily weight bearing aerobic activity
- Weight training (the ACSM recommends 10–12 reps, 2 sets 2 times weekly)
- Vitamin D (well balanced diet and adequate exposure to sunlight)
- Estrogen replacement therapy (for some women, especially post-menopausal women)

Other Hypokinetic Conditions

One out of two Americans will have a mental health disorder at some point in his or her life (Surgeon General's Report on Physical Activity and Health, 1996).

Insomnia—which is often stress related. Fifty-two percent of Americans report regular exercise helps them sleep better (Corbin, 1997).

Depression—Thirty-three percent of inactive adults report being depressed (Corbin and Lindsey, 1997). Depression can be a stress-related condition and is experienced by many adults.

Type A personality—exercise helps work out stress from a hectic life.

Prevention

- Exercise plus a prudent diet contributes to weight loss or weight management in most people.
- Exercise enhances weight loss and weight management by burning calories, speeding

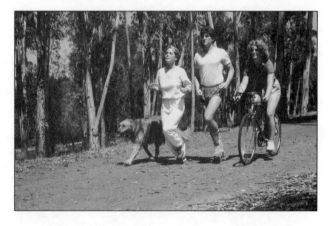

up metabolism, building muscle tissue and balancing appetite with energy expenditure.

- Evidence exists that regular activity and good physical fitness reduce the risk of hypokinetic diseases (Corbin, 1997).

- Leading public health officials have suggested that: "Physical activity is related to the health of all Americans. It has the ability to reduce directly the risk for several major chronic diseases. Physical activity may produce the shortcut we in public health have been seeking for the control of chronic diseases, much like immunization has facilitated progress against infectious diseases" (Corbin, 1997).

- Exercise and fitness can be a significant contributor to disease and illness prevention (Corbin, 1997).

- Regular exercise is effective in alleviating symptoms of diseases as well as rehabilitation after illness with diabetes, back pain and heart attack (Corbin, 1997).

- Regular exercise reduces the risk of death, regardless of cause (Corbin, 1997).

- "In fact, the national pattern of physical inactivity, in combination with the dietary patterns…ranks with tobacco use among the leading preventable contributors to death for Americans—well ahead of the contributions of infectious diseases" (Corbin, 1997).

- In 1995 the Centers for Disease Control and the American College of Sports Medicine issued recommendations for physical activity and public health that established a "strong link between regular physical activity and good health and wellness."

- For every minute exercised, you can expect to increase life expectancy by one to two minutes (Rosato, 1994).

References

American College of Sports Medicine (ACSM).

American Heart Association. 1995.

Bishop, A. *Step up to Wellness, A Stage-Based Approach*. Boston, MA: Allyn and Bacon 1999.

Corbin, L. and Lindsey. *Concepts of Physical Fitness*. 9th ed. Dubuque, IA: Brown and Benchmark 1997.

Donatelle, R. and Davis, L. *Access to Health* 4th ed. Boston, MA: Allyn and Bacon 1996.

Greenberg, J. et al. *Physical Fitness and Wellness* 2nd ed. Boston, MA: Allyn and Bacon 1998.

Hafen, B. et al. *First Aid for Colleges and Universities* 7th ed. Boston, MD: Allyn and Bacon 1999.

Harvard Alumni Study. 1986. http://www.osteo.org/osteo.html

National Center for Health Statistics.

National Institute of Health Publication. 1997. Sixth Report on the Joint National Committee on Prevention, Detection, Evaluation and Treatment of High Blood Pressure.

Paffenbarger, R. et al. "Physical Activity and Physical Fitness as Determinants of Health and Longevity." C. Bouchard et al. *Exercise Fitness and Health*. Champaign, IL: Human Kinetics Publishers 1990.

Payne, H. *Understanding Your Health* 4th ed. St. Louis, MO: Mosby 1995.

Rosato, F. *Fitness to Wellness: The Physical Connection* 3rd ed. Minneapolis: West 1994.

Surgeon General's Report on Physical Activity and Health. 1996.

Texas A&M University Human Nutrition Conference. 1998.

University of California, Berkley. November, 1990. Wellness Letter.

Contacts

American Heart Association
http://www.americanheart.org
American Medical Association
http://www.ama-assn.org

Notebook Activities

AHA Health Risk Awareness
Self-Assessment of Cardiovascular Fitness
Healthy Back Test
Body Fat Percentage
Blood Pressure Reading

■ AHA Health Risk Awareness

Take this quick quiz to find out!

You can reduce your risk of heart attack and brain attack (stroke). Start by becoming aware of your risk factors—the personal characteristics and habits that increase your chances of developing heart disease or stroke. Some you can't change or control; some you can by making a few changes in your daily habits.

Take charge of your health!

Use this quiz to learn where to focus your efforts. Then, work with your doctor to reduce, control or prevent as many risk factors as you can. Your heart and brain will thank you for taking care of yourself…
…and so will your loved ones.

Check all boxes either yes or no.

Your AGE may increase your risk if…
- ☐ Yes ☐ No You are a man over 45 years old.
- ☐ Yes ☐ No You are a woman over 55 years old, or you have passed menopause or had your ovaries removed.

Your FAMILY HISTORY may increase your risk if…
- ☐ Yes ☐ No You have a close blood relative who had a heart attack before age 55 (if father or brother) or before age 65 (if mother or sister).
- ☐ Yes ☐ No You have a close blood relative who had a brain attack (stroke).

Cigarette and tobacco SMOKE increases your risk if…
- ☐ Yes ☐ No You smoke, or live or work with people who smoke every day.

Your total CHOLESTEROL and HDL cholesterol levels may increase your risk if…
- ☐ Yes ☐ No Your total cholesterol level is 240 mg/dL or higher.
- ☐ Yes ☐ No Your HDL ("good") cholesterol level is less than 35 mg/dL.
- ☐ Yes ☐ No You don't know your total cholesterol or HDL levels.
- ☐ Yes ☐ No Your blood pressure is 140/90 mm Hg or higher, or you have been told that your blood pressure is too high.
- ☐ Yes ☐ No You don't know what your blood pressure is.

PHYSICAL INACTIVITY may increase your risk if…
- ☐ Yes ☐ No You get less than a total of 30 minutes of physical activity on at least 3 days per week.

Excess BODYWEIGHT may increase your risk if…
- ☐ Yes ☐ No You are 20 pounds or more overweight.

DIABETES increases your risk if…
- ☐ Yes ☐ No You have diabetes or need medicine to control your blood sugar.

Your MEDICAL HISTORY may increase your risk if…
- ☐ Yes ☐ No You have coronary artery disease, or you have had a heart attack.
- ☐ Yes ☐ No A doctor said you have carotid artery disease, or you have had a stroke.
- ☐ Yes ☐ No You have an abnormal heartbeat.

If you or someone you know has experienced stroke firsthand, please call the AHA's *Stroke Connection* "Warmline" 1-800-553-6321.

■ Self-Assessment of Cardiovascular Fitness

Once you've been exercising regularly for several weeks, you might want to assess your cardiovascular fitness level. Find a local track, typically one-quarter mile per lap, to perform your test. You may either run/walk for 1.5 miles and measure how long it takes to reach that distance, or run/walk for 12 minutes and determine the distance you covered in that time. Use the chart below to estimate your cardiovascular fitness level based upon your age and gender. Note that females have lower standards for each fitness category because of their higher levels of essential fat.

	1.5-Mile Run (min:sec)		12-Minute Run (miles)	
Age*	Female (min:sec)	Male (min:sec)	Female (miles)	Male (miles)
Good				
15–30	<12:00	<10:00	>1.5	>1.7
31–50	<13:30	<11:30	>1.4	>1.5
51–70	<16:00	<14:00	>1.2	>1.3
Adequate for most activities				
15–30	<13:30	<11:50	>1.4	>1.5
31–50	<15:00	<13:00	>1.3	>1.4
51–70	<17:30	<15:30	>1.1	>1.3
Borderline				
15–30	<15:00	<13:00	>1.3	>1.4
31–50	<16:30	<14:30	>1.2	>1.3
51–70	<19:00	<17:00	>1.0	>1.2
Need extra work on cardiovascular fitness				
15–30	>17:00	>15:00	<1.2	<1.3
31–50	>18:30	>16:30	<1.1	<1.2
51–70	>21:00	>19:00	<0.9	<1.0

Please list the date, location and amount of time it took you to complete 1.5 miles _____

_____

or

Please list the date, location and distance you traveled in 12 minutes _____

_____

*Cardiovascular fitness declines with age.

…If you are now at the Good level, your emphasis should be on maintaining this level for the rest of your life. If you are now at lower levels, you should set realistic goals for improvement.

■ Healthy Back Test

These tests are among the ones used by physicians and therapists to make differential diagnoses of back problems. You and your partner can use them to determine if you have muscle tightness that may make you "at risk" for back problems. Discontinue any of these tests if they produce pain or numbness, or tingling sensations in the back, hips, or legs. Experiencing any of these sensations may be an indication that you have a low back problem that requires diagnosis by your physician. Partners should use great caution in applying force. Be gentle and listen to your partner's feedback.

Test 1—Back to Wall

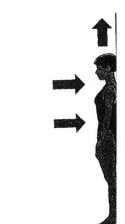

Stand with your back against a wall, with head, heels, shoulders, and calves of legs touching the wall as shown in the diagram. Try to flatten your neck and the hollow of your back by pressing your buttocks down against the wall. Your partner should just be able to place a hand in the space between the wall and the small of your back.

- If this space is greater than the thickness of his/her hand, you probably have lordosis with shortened lumbar and hip flexor muscles.

Test 2—Straight Leg Lift

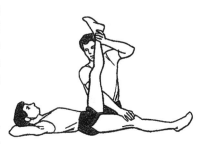

Lie on your back with hands behind your neck. The partner on your left should stabilize your right leg by placing his/her right hand on the knee. With the left hand, your partner should grasp the left ankle and raise your left leg as near to a right angle as possible. In this position (as shown in the diagram), your lower back should be in contact with the floor. Your right leg should remain straight and on the floor throughout the test.

- If your left leg bends at the knee, short hamstring muscles are indicated. If your back arches and/or your right leg does not remain flat on the floor, short lumbar muscles or hip flexor muscles (or both) are indicated. Repeat the test on the opposite side. (Both sides must pass in order to pass the test).

Test 3—Thomas Test

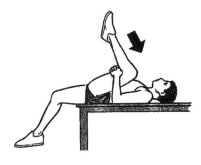

Lie on your back on a table or bench with your right leg extended beyond the edge of the table (approximately one-third of the thigh off the table). Bring your left knee to your chest and pull the thigh down tightly with your hands. Your lower back should remain flat against the table as shown in the diagram. Your right thigh should remain on the table.

- If your right thigh lifts off the table while the left knee is hugged to the chest, a tight hip flexor (iliopsoas) on that side is indicated. Repeat on the opposite side. (Both sides must pass in order to pass the test.)

Test 4—Ely's Test

Lie prone; flex right knee. Partner gently pushes right heel toward the buttocks. Stop when resistance is felt or when partner expresses discomfort.

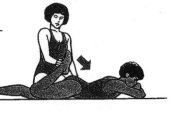

- If pelvis leaves the floor or hip flexes or knee fails to bend freely (135 degrees) or heel fails to touch buttocks, there is tightness in the quadriceps muscles. Repeat with left leg. (Both sides must pass to pass the test.)

Test 5—Ober's Test

Lie on left side with left leg flexed 90 degrees at the hip and 90 degrees at the knee. Partner places right hip in neutral position (no flexion) and right knee in 90-degree flexion; partner then allows the weight of the leg to lower it toward the floor.

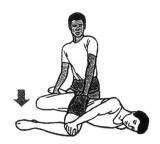

- If there is no tightness in the iliotibial band (fascia and muscles on lateral side of leg), the knee touches the floor without pain and the test is passed. Repeat on the other side. (Both sides must pass in order to pass the test.)

Test 6—Press-Up (Straight Arm)

Perform the press-up.

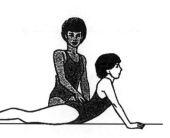

- If you can press to a straight-arm position, keeping your pubis in contact with the floor, and if your partner determines that the arch in your back is a continuous curve (not just a sharp angle at the lumbosacral joint), then there is adequate flexibility in spinal extension.

Test 7—Knee Roll

Lie supine with both knees and hips flexed 90 degrees, arms extended to the sides at shoulder level. Keep the knees and hips in that position and lower them to the floor on the right and then on the left.

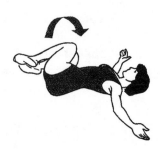

- If you can accomplish this and still keep your shoulders in contact with the floor, then you have adequate rotation in the spine, especially at the lumbar and thoracic junction. (You must pass both sides in order to pass the test.)

Healthy Back Ratings

Classification	Number of Tests Passed
Excellent	7
Very good	6
Good	5
Fair	4
Poor	1-3

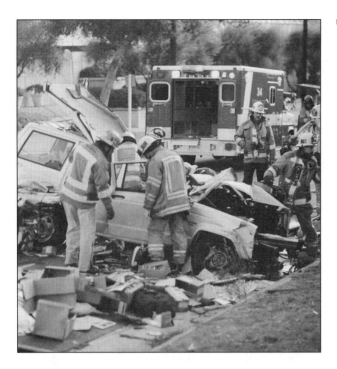

Chapter Four

Safety Awareness

"Cruelty might be very human, and it might be very cultural, but it's not acceptable"

—Jodie Foster, Academy Award acceptance
speech for her role in *The Accused*

OBJECTIVES

Students will be able to:

- Identify the four classes of accidents

- Identify risks associated with drowsy driving

- Identify elements of a crime

- Identify steps in preventing a sexual assault

- Become aware of the prevalence of acquaintance rape

- Become aware of the prevalence of domestic violence

- Identify organizations that provide assistance to victims of violent crime

The purpose of this chapter is to provide information to help students make informed choices on personal safety and awareness issues. Being aware of possible hazardous situations may prevent accidents from occurring and possibly save lives.

The National Safety Council defines an accident as "that occurrence in a sequence of events which usually produces unintended injury, death, or property damage" (Bever, 1995). Accidents are the fifth leading cause of death in the United States after heart disease, cancer, stroke, or chronic obstructive pulmonary diseases. For people between the ages of 1 and 38, accidents are the leading cause of death. In 1997 there were 93,800 accidental deaths overall, and 19,300,000 disabling injuries (National Safety Council, 1998).

There are four classes of accidents:

1. Motor vehicle accidents
2. Home-related accidents
3. Work accidents
4. Public accidents

Risks and Hazards

According to the National Safety Council, a *hazard* is defined as a condition or set of conditions, which have the potential to produce injury and/or property damage. The probability that a hazard will be activated and produce injury/property damage is the definition of *risk*.

Hazards are generally the same for everyone, but risks tend to be more of an individual choice. What is a risk for some may not be a risk for others. In determining the safety of risks, one must measure the risk and judge the acceptability of that particular risk. The use of alcohol and other drugs as well as attitudes and emotions play a role in personal safety. Thrill seeking, stress, anger, and inattentiveness can also contribute to the likelihood of becoming involved in an accident.

Classes of Accidents

Motor Vehicle

The leading cause of accidental death is motor vehicle accidents, killing over 40,000 people annually and injuring two million people per year. Some common causes of motor vehicle accidents are speeding, failure to yield the right of way, driving while intoxicated, disregarding traffic signals and fatigue.

Speeding is one of the main factors contributing to motor vehicle accidents. The faster you are traveling, the less time you have to react, the longer it takes to stop. It reduces a driver's ability to steer safely around objects and causes a harder impact.

Failure to yield right of way whether entering an expressway, busy street or changing lanes, is the cause of many accidents, some which can be fatal.

DWI—alcohol is responsible for almost fifty percent of motor vehicle accidents and is the leading cause of motor vehicle fatalities (National Highway Traffic Safety Administration, 1998). These accidents and fatalities are one hundred percent avoidable by choosing not to drink and drive.

Disregarding Traffic Signals—is one of the major causes for motor vehicle accidents from the standpoint that when a person runs through a red light, they are usually speeding to try to "beat the light," not realizing the impact they will cause to another vehicle.

Driver Drowsiness—Fatigue on the road can be a killer. It happens frequently on long trips, especially long night drives. According to the National Highway Traffic Safety Administration (NHTSA), drowsy driving accounts for approximately 56,000 accidents each year, injuring 40,000 and producing 1,550 fatalities. In some cases, it is more dangerous to drive when you are drowsy than intoxicated. The majority of these accidents involve male drivers less than 30 years of age. To prevent this problem, it is best to choose not to drive if you are feeling fatigued, in planning a trip it is best to be rested.

The National Sleep Foundation offers these tips for staying awake while driving (Travisano, 1998):

- Get a good night's sleep
- Schedule regular stops
- Drive with a companion
- Avoid alcohol
- Avoid medications that may cause drowsiness

If anti-fatigue measures don't work, of course the best solution is sleep. If no motels are in sight and you are within one to two hours of your destination, pull off the road in a safe area and take a short twenty to thirty minute nap.

Bicycle Safety

According to the National Safety Council, bicycle related head injuries in 1997, resulted in 813 deaths and accounted for 567,000 emergency room visits. Wearing a helmet reduces the risk of serious head injuries by as much as 85 percent and the risk of brain injury by as much as 88 percent (NHTSA, 1998). Helmets have also been shown to reduce injuries to upper and mid-face by 65 percent.

If each rider wore a helmet an estimated 500 bicycle related fatalities and 151,000 non-fatal head injuries would be prevented each year (Journal of American Medical Association, 1998).

Helmet Laws

According to the Bicycle Helmet Safety Institute, by early 1999 15 states and more than 65 local governments had enacted some form of bicycle helmet legislation, most dealing with children or adolescents.

Ensuring that helmets provide real protection U.S. Consumer Product Safety Commission (CPSC) issued a new safety standard for bike helmets in 1999. The new standard ensures that bike helmets will adequately protect the head and that chin-straps will be strong enough to prevent the helmet from coming off in a crash, collision or fall. All bike helmets in the U.S. must meet the CPSC standard.

Prevention

According to the National Center for Injury Prevention and Control:

- Wear your helmet correctly. A helmet should fit snuggly and not rock forward, backward, or side-to-side.
- Only buy a helmet if it meets or exceeds CPSC standards.
- Obey all traffic laws! Bicycles must adhere to all motor vehicle traffic laws.
- When riding at night, you must have a white front reflector or bright headlight and red rear reflector.

Home Accidents

Falls

There are over 25,000 deaths each year in the U.S. that occur at home, as well as almost a million disabling injuries. The leading cause of death due to home injuries is falls, resulting in over 9,000 deaths per year. The age groups most prone to death from falls are the elderly and the very young, 0-4 years old (National Safety Council, 1998).

Poisoning

The second leading cause of death in the home is poisoning. Poisonings account for almost 7,000 deaths annually. Included in this category are deaths from drugs and other medicines, which could explain why the 25-44 year age group represents over 4,000 deaths per year. Children under 5 years of age are especially susceptible to household poisons, such as cleaning agents and medications.

Poisoning by gases and vapors causes an average of 400 deaths each year. The primary cause of gas poisoning is carbon monoxide (odorless and colorless gas) due to incomplete combustion involving heating equipment, cooking stoves, and motor vehicle exhaust. To avoid carbon monoxide poisoning in the homes always have your heating system checked annually for leaks and proper ventilation.

Fires and Burns

Fires and burns account for between 3,000-4,000 deaths each year and are the third leading cause of unintentional death in the home (NSC, 1998). The U.S. has more fire deaths each year than any other industrialized country. According to the U.S. Fire Administration, cigarette smoking is the leading cause of residential fire deaths.

Three factors can be effective in preventing injuries and fatalities from fires:

1. Take responsibility and view fire as a personal threat. We sometimes feel that fires happen to "someone else," not us.
2. Take precautions and preventative measures, such as installing smoke detectors, carbon monoxide detectors, and fire extinguishers in the home.
3. Implement a plan of action for escaping a fire to save valuable time as well as your life.

Work Accidents

The National Safety Council estimates that over 5,000 people each year die as a result of work-related accidents and almost 4,000,000 are injured. The Occupational Safety and Health Act was passed in 1970 to assure safe working conditions for every man and woman in the U.S. The Occupational Safety and Health Administration (OSHA), is the governing body established to enforce safety rules and regulations.

The leading cause of occupational death is *motor vehicle accidents*. According to the National Safety Council, motor vehicle accidents account for over 20 percent of the occupational deaths, which primarily involve the transportation industry; 14 percent of the deaths are due to *assaults on the job* (workplace violence), 9 percent are due to *falls*, and 9 percent come from being *struck by an object*.

Occupational illnesses are conditions caused by repeated exposure to factors associated with employment, such as *repetitive strain injury* (RSI), or repeated trauma. An example of RSI, *Carpal Tunnel Syndrome* (CTS) is inflammation in the tendons of the wrist, damaging nerves in the hand and can be caused by typing, computer use, or any repeated use of the hands. Certain occupations pose a higher risk for CTS, such as computer technicians, clerical workers, electricians, carpenters, and those in the manufacturing field.

Public Accidents

These accidents include deaths in public places and non-motor vehicle accidents. Fatalities consist of water and air transportation accidents, railroad accidents, recreational boating and drowning fatalities, sports injuries and deaths, as well as fatalities as a result of natural disasters. Water, air, and railroad transportation deaths account for over 1,500 deaths annually (NSC, 1998).

According to data from the United States Coast Guard, deaths associated with recreational boating average about 700 each year. Injuries associated with Personal Watercraft (PWC), have increased, accounting for over 1,800 deaths annually.

Sports Injuries—Data from the National Safety Council indicates that basketball and bicycle riding account for more than half a million emergency room visits each year. The National Safety Council also estimates there were 1,500 swimming fatalities reported in 1997.

Tornadoes are the most destructive of all storms, causing almost 90 deaths each year. According to data from the National Climatic Data Center (NCDC), Texas has the greatest number of tornadoes, with 132 during an average year.

Over the last 38 years, *lightning* has accounted for an average of 89 deaths per year according to the NCDC. States with the greatest number of lightning deaths during these years were Florida, Texas, and North Carolina.

Personal Safety

Personal safety is an issue that affects our everyday lives, regardless of who we are or where we live, and it is essential to take certain precautions for protection. Being aware of surroundings and learning to avoid certain situations can prevent many negative consequences.

In order for a crime to take place, three elements must exist:

1. The ability of the criminal
2. The desire of the criminal
3. An opportunity for the crime to be committed

As individuals, we can only control one of the above elements, the most important—opportunity. If the criminal does not have the opportunity to commit a crime, it certainly diminishes the likelihood of the crime actually taking place. There are no guarantees, but by being more aware as individuals, some hazardous situation can be avoided.

According to the Bureau of Justice Statistics (BJS) 1997 National Crime Victimization Survey, persons 12 years of age or older living in the U.S. experienced approximately 34.8 million crimes.

- 74% (25.8 million) property crimes
- 25% (8.6 million) crimes of violence
- 1% personal thefts

According to the BJS, there are a few basic safety tips and precautions to lower your risk of becoming a victim.

Home
- Always keep doors and windows locked.
- Have adequate lighting around home or apartment (notify apt. manager).
- Do not open door to strangers—ask for credentials from maintenance or repair personnel.
- Do not give personal information over the telephone.
- Prepare records of personal items.

Campus
- Avoid walking alone.
- Do not leave personal possessions unattended.
- Always notice other people—make eye contact.
- Avoid taking shortcuts through campus.
- Do not walk like a victim. Walk like you are on a mission.
- Always be aware of your surroundings.
- Trust your instincts. If someone or something makes you feel uncomfortable, get out of the situation.

Car
- Keep doors and windows locked.
- Always park in well-lighted areas.
- If being followed, do not go home. Go to a police station or well-populated area.
- Be aware of your surroundings at all times.

Sexual Assault

Rape is not about sex, it's about power. Most rape victims are women, but that does not exclude men as victims. It is estimated that only about 10 percent of rape cases are reported and that in one out of seven reported rapes, the victim is a male.

Forcible rape is comprised of three elements: the use of force (not necessarily physical), absence of consent by the victim, and penile/vaginal penetration. Rape can happen to anyone at any age. Ages of reported cases range from 6 months to 90 years old with the majority of victims under the age of 25 and the majority of their attackers also under the age of 25 (Weinberg, 1994).

Most rapists plan their attack by familiarizing themselves with the victim's surroundings. In all rape cases, the attacker has the advantage from a surprise standpoint. Being aware of your surroundings and avoiding certain situations may help prevent sexual assaults or any violent crime from occurring.

The Department of Justice estimates that for every sexual assault, there are at least two attempts made on someone. Studies by the Department of Justice have shown that women who used physical resistance at the beginning of the attack were two times more likely to escape rape than those that did not resist. Although choosing to resist increases your chance of injuries, you will have a higher probability of avoiding rape.

Active resistance can be used in an attack situation. Examples can be: screaming, running, and using physical force. If attacked, there are three questions that you should ask yourself:

1. What am I capable of doing?
2. What is my attacker capable of doing?
3. Where am I? (location, etc.)

Your response to an attack depends on the answers to these questions. Are you capable of using physical force? If so, then do it. Learning basic self-defense can be extremely helpful in gaining self-confidence.

How you respond to the situation has a lot to do with where you are, i.e. in a mall parking lot, or in a deserted park in the middle of nowhere. The best defense against an attack is to have a plan and an idea of what you would do if you were ever in a situation which calls for a response. It is a good idea to have several plans to choose from because no two situations are alike. What works in one situation may not work in another. There are no guarantees!

Passive resistance could be effective in some situations. Examples of passive resistance would be verbal persuasion, pleading or submission. This sometimes can be helpful in regaining your stability and possibly giving you a chance to think through the situation and plan a defense. However, research has shown that passive resistance is not as effective as active resistance and does not seem to reduce the chance of victim injury (Bever, 1995).

Prevalence

The frequency of occurrence for rape and sexual assault is astounding. According to the Rape Abuse and Incest National Network (RAINN, 1999):

- In the U.S., a woman is sexually assaulted every two minutes (U.S. Department of Justice)
- 307,000 women were victims of rape, attempted rape or sexual assault (1996 National Crime Victimization Survey)
- In 1996, only 31 percent of rapes and sexual assaults were reported, less than one in every three
- 68 percent of rape victims knew their assailant (Violence Against Women Bureau of Justice Statistics)
- 28 percent of victims are raped by husbands or boyfriends
- 35 percent of victims are raped by acquaintances
- 5 percent of victims are raped by relatives

According to the U.S. Department of Justice—Violence Against Women (1994).

- 1 in every 4 rapes takes place in a public place
- 29 percent of female victims reported the victim was a stranger
- 45 percent of rapists were under the influence of alcohol
- In 29 percent of rapes the offender used a weapon
- One in two rape victims are under the age of 18

According to the National Crime Victimization Survey (1996):

- 9 out of 10 rape victims are women. 1995— 32,130 males age 12 and older were victims of rape or attempted rapes.
- Teens 16 to 19 were three and one half times more likely than the general population to be victims of rape or attempted rape.

Ways to Reduce Risks of Sexual Assault

- When at a party or club, don't leave beverages unattended or accept a drink from someone you don't know.
- When you go to a party or club, go with friends and leave with friends.
- Be aware of your surroundings at all times.
- Don't allow yourself to be isolated with someone you don't know.
- Know the level of intimacy you want in a relationship and state your limits.
- Trust your instincts.

Steps to Take if Rape Occurs

- Go to a friend's house or call someone you know to come over. You do not need to be alone!
- DO NOT shower or make any attempt to clean yourself, do not change clothes or remove any physical evidence of the attack.
- Call your local Rape Crisis Center for assistance and counseling. A counselor can also accompany you to the hospital.
- Seek immediate medical attention and notify the police.

Acquaintance Rape/Intimate Violence

According to the Bureau of Justice Statistics, in 1996 women experienced an estimated 840,000 rapes or sexual assaults at the hands of someone intimate. Women ages 16 to 24 experience the highest per capita rates of intimate violence (intimate is defined as current or former spouse, boyfriends and girlfriends). In almost 80 percent of cases involving sexual assault or rape, the victim knew the attacker. It is estimated that approximately one in four female college students have

been sexually assaulted or an attempt of sexual assault has been made on them since the age of 14.

The Bureau of Justice Statistics estimates about three million violent crimes occur each year in which the offenders have been drinking alcohol at the time of the offense. Two-thirds of victims who suffered violence by an intimate reported that alcohol had been a factor. Approximately 31 percent of stranger victimizations were alcohol related.

Domestic Violence

According to the Surgeon General, domestic violence is the leading cause of injury to women between the ages of 15 and 44, approximately 70 percent of men who abuse their female partners, also abuse their children. Every day in America, intimate male partners kill at least 4 women, and more than 50 percent of women, in the United States are battered at sometime in their lives.

Organizations

Most communities have a Rape Crisis Center as well as centers for domestic violence. National Information Hotlines are also available.

For help contact:

Rape Abuse & Incest National Network
1-800-656-HOPE
http://www.rainn.org

National Coalition against Domestic Violence
P.O. Box 34103
Washington, D.C 20043-4103
202-638-6388

National Coalition against Sexual Assault
P.O. Box 21378
Washington, D.C. 20009
202-483-7165

VOICES in Action
P.O. Box 148309
Chicago, IL 60614
312-327-1500

National Domestic Violence Hotline
1-800-799-SAFE

National Victim Center
1-800-FYI-CALL

References

Bever, David L. *Safety—A Personal Focus.* 3rd ed. St. Louis, Mo: Mosby Year Book, 1992.

Bureau of Justice Statistics, U.S. Department of Justice, 1997 National Crime Victimization Survey.

Koop, C. Everett, M.D. *U.S. Surgeon General's Report.* U.S. Public Health Service, 1988.

National Coalition Against Domestic Violence, 1989.

National Highway Traffic Safety Administration, http://www.nhtsa.dot.gov.

National Safety Council: *Accident Facts™, 1998 Edition*, Itasca, IL 1998

Rape Abuse and Incest National Network, RAINN, http://www.rainn.org

Stout, K.A. Intimate Femicide: A National Demographic Overview. *Journal of Interpersonal Violence*, 6(4), 1991, pp. 476–485.

Texas Council on Family Violence, "Statistics on Domestic Violence." 1997. Austin TX.

Travisano, Jim. The Dangers of Drowsy Driving, *Current Health 2*, March 1998

Weinberg, Carol. *The Complete Handbook of College Women.* (New York: New York University Press, 1994.)

Williams, Brian K. and Sharon M. Knight. *Healthy for Life—Wellness and the Art of Living.* Pacific Grove, CA: Brooks/Cole Publishing Company, 1997.

Notebook Activity

Checklist of Rape Prevention Strategies

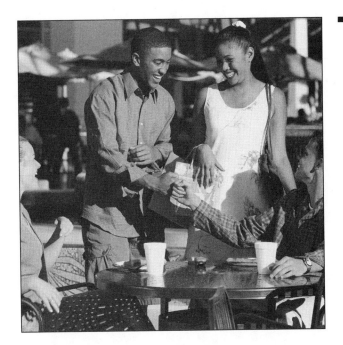

Chapter Five

Sexuality

"A healthy attitude is contagious, but don't wait to catch it from others. Be a carrier."

—source unknown

OBJECTIVES

Students will be able to:

- correctly identify structures of the female and male sexual anatomy.

- list three different types of STIs.

- differentiate between the STIs and list three ways to decrease the risk of contraction.

- identify methods and their effectiveness in the prevention of sexually transmitted infections and pregnancy.

- name and describe the stages of the menstrual cycle.

- be able to explain the female and male reproductive process.

- identify the options in the case of an unplanned pregnancy.

The purpose of this chapter is to familiarize students with the female and male anatomy and gender-specific cycles. Material will be presented detailing various sexually transmitted infections (STIs), the health risks associated with contraction of STIs and various preventative measures and techniques in STIs and pregnancy. Additional information will be presented on parenthood and the options that exist when pregnancy prevention is not effective.

Anatomy

Female Sexual Anatomy, Physiology and Response

The female anatomy consists of multiple integral parts both externally and internally. (See Figure 5.1) The *vulva* includes visible external genitalia. The *mons pubis* is the soft fatty tissue covering the pubic symphysis (joint of the pubic bones). This area is covered with pubic hair that begins growing during puberty. The *labia majora* include two longitudinal folds of skin that extend on both sides of the vulva and serve as protection for the inner

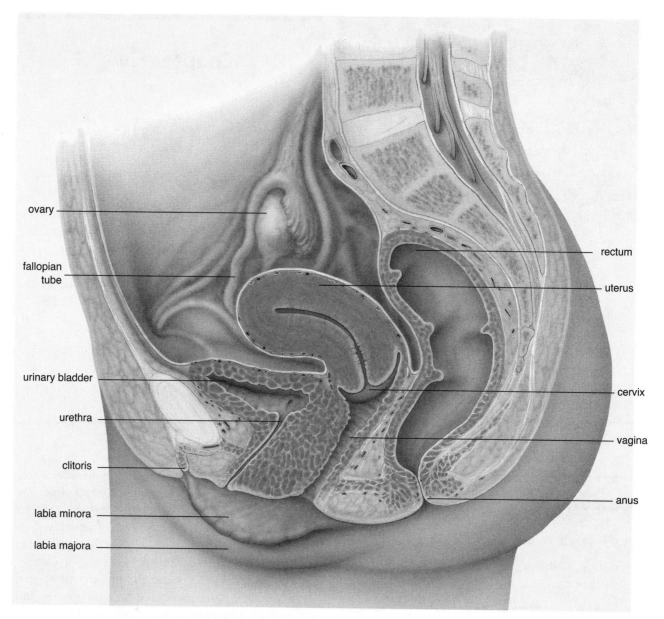

ovary

fallopian tube

urinary bladder

urethra

clitoris

labia minora

labia majora

rectum

uterus

cervix

vagina

anus

FIGURE 5.1 Organs of the female reproductive system.

parts of the vulva. The *labia minora* are the delicate inner folds of skin that enclose the urethral opening and the vagina. These skin flaps, which contain sweat and oil glands, extensive blood vessels and nerve endings, are hairless and sensitive to touch. When sexually stimulated, the labia minora swell and darken. The *clitoris* is usually the most sensitive part of the female genitalia. The clitoris consists of erectile tissue, which becomes engorged with blood, resulting in swelling during sexual arousal that enables it to double in size. The *clitoral hood* consists of inner lips, which join to form a soft fold of skin, or hood, covering and connecting to the clitoris. The *urethra* is approximately 2.5 cm below the clitoris and functions as the opening for urine to be excreted from the bladder. Because the urethra is located close to the vaginal opening, some irritation may result from vigorous or prolonged sexual activity. The most common problem associated with this is the development of urinary tract infections. The *vagina* is located between the urethral opening and the anus. The *hymen* is the small membrane within the vaginal opening that is believed to tear during initial intercourse, with tampon use, while riding a horse or other various types of athletic activities. The only function of the hymen is to protect the vaginal tissues early in life. The *perineum* is the smooth skin located between the labia minora and the anus. During childbirth this area may tear or be cut (episiotomy) as the newborn passes out of the vagina. The *anal canal* is located just behind the perineum and allows for elimination of solid waste. The anal canal is approximately an inch long with two sphincter muscles, which open and close like valves. Internally, just past the vagina, is the cervix, which connects the vagina and the uterus. (See Figure 5.2) The *uterus* is the hollow, pear-shaped mus-

cular organ about the size of a fist when a female is not pregnant. This is the organ in which the fetus develops during pregnancy. The upper expanded portion is referred to as the fundus and the lower constricted part is the cervix. On each side of the uterus there is a *fallopian tube*, which is quite narrow and approximately four inches in length. Because of the narrow passageway within these tubes, infection and scarring may cause fertility problems. Most women have a right and a left fallopian tube. These tubes extend from the ovaries to the uterus and transport mature ovum. Fertilization usually takes place within the fallopian tubes. The opening between the fallopian tube and the uterus is only about as wide as a needle. On each end of the fallopian tubes are the *ovaries*, where eggs are produced and released usually once a month. Each ovary is about the size of a large olive.

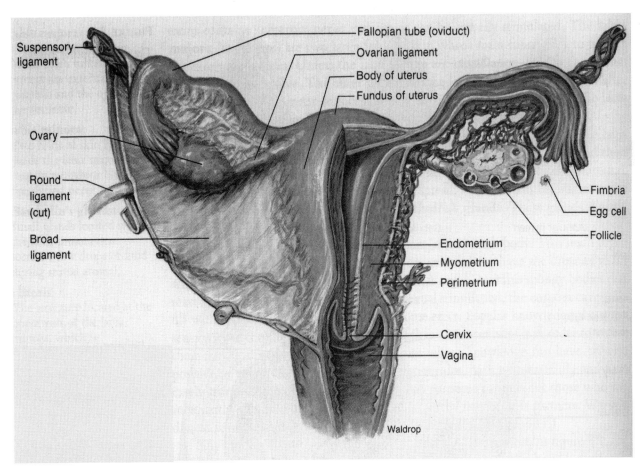

From *Sexuality: Insights and Issues*, Third Edition. Copyright © 1993 by Jerrold Greenberg, Clint Buess, and Kathleen D. Mullen. Reprinted by permission of the authors.

FIGURE 5.2 An anterior view of the female reproductive organs showing the relationship of the ovaries, uterine tubes, uterus, cervix, and vagina.

At birth, a female's ovaries contain 40,000 to 400,000 immature ova, of which approximately 450 will mature and be released during the reproductive years. The ovaries also produce the hormones estrogen and progesterone, both of which help regulate the menstrual cycle (Sloane, 1993).

The female *sexual response* consists of four phases: excitement, plateau, orgasm, and resolution. During the excitement phase vaginal lubrication begins and the vagina, clitoris, labia majora and minora all fill with blood. The nipples swell and there is increased tension in many voluntary muscles. During plateau, the vaginal opening usually decreases in diameter due to swelling, the uterus usually increases in size and the labia majora and minora become more swollen and engorged. During an orgasm the muscles of the vaginal wall undergo rhythmic contractions. The number of contractions may range from three to as many as twelve. Involuntary contraction of other muscles may take place as well. During resolution blood rapidly returns to the rest of the body from the vagina, clitoris, labia majora and minora, resulting in reduced swelling. At this time the breasts also return to their original size (Sloane, 1993).

Male Sexual Anatomy, Physiology and Response

The external male sexual structures include the penis and scrotum. The *penis* is an organ through which semen and urine pass, and is structured into three main sections: the root, the shaft and the

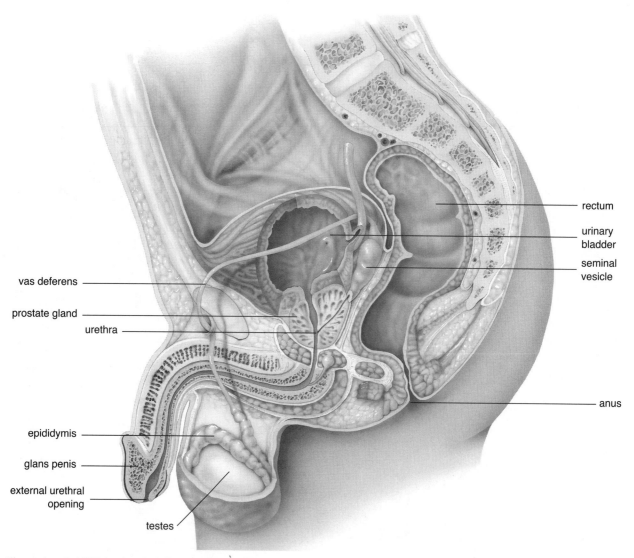

Illustration © 1997 Anatomical Chart Co., Skokie, IL

FIGURE 5.3 Side view of the male reproductive organs.

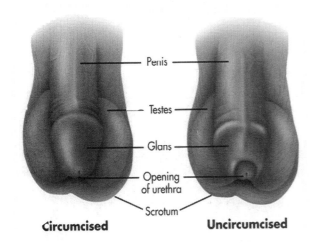

Penis
Testes
Glans
Opening
of urethra
Scrotum

Circumcised **Uncircumcised**

FIGURE 5.4 External male genitalia.

glans penis. (See Figure 5.3) The root attaches the penis within the pelvic cavity at the base, while the shaft, or the tube-shaped body of the penis, hangs freely. The *glans penis* is covered by a loose portion of tissue called the *foreskin*, which may be removed during a surgery known as circumcision. A penis without foreskin is circumcised, while one with the foreskin intact is uncircumcised (See Figure 5.4). At the base of the glans is a rim known as the corona. On the underside is a triangular area of highly sensitive skin called the frenulum, which attaches the glans to the foreskin (Strong, 1996). The glans penis is the soft, fleshy enlarged tissue at the end of the shaft, with the urethral opening at the tip (Moglia et al., 1997). The *scrotum* is the pouch of skin, which hangs from the root of the penis and holds the two testicles. Covered sparsely with hair, the scrotum is divided in the middle by a ridge of skin, showing the separation of the testes. The surface changes of the scrotum help maintain a moderately constant temperature within the testes (~93 degrees F), which is important for maintaining good sperm production (Strong, et al., 1996). The male internal sexual structures include the testes, epididymus, vas deferens, seminal vesicles, prostate and Cowper's glands. The *testes* are the reproductive ball-shaped glands inside the scrotum which are also referred to as testicles. Sperm and hormone production are the two main functions of the testes (Moglia, et al., 1997). Sperm are formed constantly,

beginning during puberty, inside the 750 feet of highly coiled thin tubes called seminiferous tubules within each testes (Moglia, et al., 1997). Between the seminiferous tubules are cells that produce sexual hormones. One such important hormone is testosterone, which stimulates the production of sperm (Moglia, et al., 1997). On top of each testis is another tightly coiled tube, the *epididymis*, where nearly mature sperm complete the maturation process (Moglia, et al., 1997). Mature sperm are stored in the epididymis until they are released during ejaculation. The *vas deferens* is a long tube through which sperm travel during ejaculation. The epididymis is connected to the *seminal vesicle* via the vas deferens, which is responsible for contracting and pushing the sperm to the seminal vesicle (Moglia, et al., 1997). Located beneath the bladder are the two small seminal vesicles, which secrete a fluid that provides nourishment as well as an environment conducive to sperm mobility. After the sperm have combined with the seminal fluid, they reach the prostate where another substance is added. A thin, milky fluid is produced by the prostate and secreted into the urethra during the time of emission of semen, which enhances the swimming environment for the sperm (Moglia, et al., 1997). Below the prostate and attached to the urethra are the two pea-sized *Cowper's glands*, responsible for depositing a lubricating fluid for sperm and a coating for the urethra (Moglia, et al., 1997). If there are sperm in the urethra from a previous ejaculation, they will mix with the Cowper's fluid and become a pre-ejaculate lubricant fluid (Moglia, et al., 1997). Ejaculation occurs at the peak of sexual excitement when the prostate muscle opens and sends the seminal fluid to the urethra where it is then forced out through the urethral opening, forming semen (Moglia, et al., 1997).

The shaft of the penis can change dramatically during *sexual arousal*. During sexual excitement, tiny muscles inside the shaft tissue called corpus spongiosum and corpus cavernosa relax and open, allowing inflow of blood (Moglia, et al., 1997). As these tissues fill with blood, the penis becomes longer, thicker and less flexible, thus resulting in an erection. Although sexual sensitivity is unique among individuals, the glans penis is particularly important in sexual arousal due to its high concentration of nerve endings (Strong, et al., 1996). When a man is either sexually aroused or cold, the testes are pulled close to the body (Strong, et al., 1996).

From *Sexuality: Insights and Issues,* Third Edition. Copyright © 1993 by Jerrold Greenberg, Clint Buess, and Kathleen D. Mullen. Reprinted by permission of the authors.

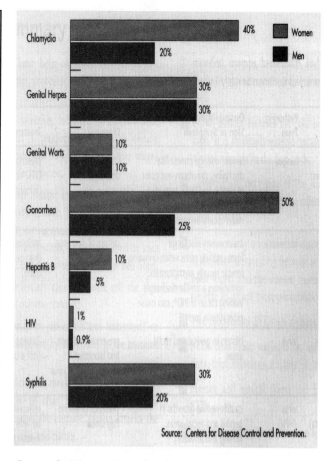

Centers for Disease Control and Prevention.

FIGURE 5.5 Rates for contracting various STIs after one heterosexual unprotected intercourse.

Sexually Transmitted Infections (STIs)

Sexually transmitted infections are transmitted during vaginal, oral, anal sexual activity or in some cases by simply touching an infected area. STIs can be transferred not only to the genitalia area, but also to the mouth, eyes, nose and other orifices of the body. Many individuals who become infected with STIs are asymptomatic (without symptoms) and thus become silent carriers. This is one of the reasons STIs have reached epidemic proportions.

Bacterial STIs

Chlamydia

Chlamydia is caused by a bacteria-like intracellular parasite called Chlamydia trachomati. Chlamydia is typically spread during vaginal, oral or anal sex and can infect other body parts such as the eyes, nose or throat where chlamydia can also be contracted. Symptoms in males include a thin, clear-whitish urethral discharge, itching or burning during urination, pain or swelling in the testes and a low-

grade fever. In females, symptoms include moderate vaginal discharge, itching or burning during urination, abdominal pain, bleeding between periods, nausea, headaches and a low-grade fever. If symptoms occur, they will typically begin one to three weeks after infection. As mentioned previously, most infected females and many infected males are asymptomatic. The long-term effects of untreated Chlamydia can include blindness after infection of the eyes and sterility in both males and females from scar tissue forming in the testicles and fallopian tubes. Chlamydia infections are the leading cause of preventable infertility and ectopic pregnancies. Most infections respond to tetracycline, doxycycline or erythromycin, but not penicillin. It is very important that all partners be treated to decrease the spread of infection as well as prevent reinfection. Chlamydia is estimated to be the most common bacterial STI in the United States, with approximately three to four million new cases occurring each year (Kassler et al., 1992). Adolescents and young adults have the highest infection rates, with an estimated six to ten percent of all college students diagnosed with this infection (Lee, 1989; Keim, et al., 1992).

Gonorrhea

Gonorrhea is caused by the bacteria called Neisseria gonorrhea. Infection is found primarily in the linings of the urethra, vagina, mouth and rectum although infection can occur in the eyes (Crowley, 1992). Symptoms in males include a foul smelling thick creamy white, yellow, or yellow-green discharge from the penis, painful urination, blood or pus in the urine and enlarged lymph nodes in the groin area. In females, the symptoms include similar discharge from the vagina, pain during urination, pelvic pain or irregular and painful menstruation. If symptoms are present, they usually occur three to five days after infection. As with Chlamydia infections, many individuals are asymptomatic (*five to 20 percent of infected males and 60 to 80 percent of females*). The long-term effects of untreated gonorrhea can cause sterility in both males and females, as a result of infection and scarring in both testicles and in the fallopian tubes. Most infections respond to penicillin, tetracycline, spectinomycin, cefixime, or ceftriaxone. It is very important that all partners be treated to decrease the spread of the infection as well as prevent reinfection.

Syphilis

Syphilis is a serious bacterial infection caused by the spirochete Treponema pallidum. Syphilis can be contracted and spread through vaginal, oral or anal sex as well as through blood and blood products. This infection can be debilitating and even fatal if left untreated. A person may be unknowingly infected with syphilis and transmit it to others. There are an estimated 120,000 new cases of syphilis in the U.S. each year (Microsoft Encarta, 1997). This disease has three stages. During the first stage, a painless sore (chancre) may appear at the point where the bacteria first entered the body, usually 10 to 90 days after infection. This sore may appear around or in the vagina, on the penis, or inside the mouth or anus. Sores inside the vagina or anus are often unnoticed and may disappear on their own if not treated, however the bacterial infection remains. The second stage occurs three

weeks to three months after the primary stage and includes flu like symptoms and possible hair loss, a rash on the palms of hands and soles of feet, as well as over the entire body. The tertiary (third stage) syphilis can appear three to ten years or more after the first and second stages. Symptoms of this stage may include skin lesions, mental deterioration, loss of balance and vision, loss of sensation, shooting pains in the legs and heart disease (Microsoft Encarta, 1997). See a physician immediately if there is any chance you have been exposed to syphilis. A simple blood test can usually determine whether or not you have the infection. However, if you become infected two to three weeks prior to testing, the blood test may not be sensitive enough to detect the antibodies. Syphilis can be treated with the proper antibiotics, most commonly penicillin injections.

There have been several resistant strains that have developed when individuals did not take the full prescription dose. *Always* take all of the antibiotics that are prescribed to you; don't save them for later or stop them just because you feel better and *never* take someone else's medication.

Viral STIs

Genital Herpes

Genital Herpes is a chronic, lifelong viral infection. Herpes can be contracted and spread through vaginal, oral or anal sex as well as skin to skin contact. Herpes simplex I (cold sores) can be transmitted to the genital region. A mother can also infect her newborn child during delivery if she has an active outbreak. Infection in the newborn can cause mental retardation, blindness or even death (Tseng, 1987). Therefore, it is important that an infected pregnant female inform her physician of the infection so that the physician can watch for an outbreak and perform a cesarean section (C-Section) if necessary. An estimated 40 million people have genital herpes (Center for Prevention Services). Each year there are approximately 500,000 new cases of symptomatic herpes (CDC.GOV). There are many more individuals who have genital herpes and are asymptomatic. The symptoms vary, and many people have no noticeable symptoms. Symptoms will most commonly occur within two to twenty days after infection. Early symptoms may include a tingling or burning sensation in the genitals, lower back pain, pain when urinating and flu-like symptoms (Center for Prevention Services, U.S. Venereal Disease Control Division). A few days later, small red bump(s) may appear in the genital area. Later, these bumps can develop into painful blisters, which then crust over, form a scab and heal. Sometimes the diagnosis can be made by physical examination alone. For testing, the physician collects a small amount of fluid from the sores to see if the herpes virus is present. It may take up to two weeks to receive the results. If no sores are present, testing may be difficult. However, a blood test does exist to determine if an individual does have the herpes virus. It is very expensive and does not indicate the location of the infection. Although herpes is a chronic, lifelong viral infection, the symptoms can be treated. Treatment of genital herpes outbreaks, especially when begun early, shortens the duration of the outbreak and reduces the severity of the symptoms (Marr, 1998). Medications used include acyclovir, famcyclovir and valacyclovir. Individuals with more than six outbreaks per year may be treated with preventative (prophylactic) suppressive therapy.

HIV/AIDS

Human Immunodeficiency Virus (HIV)/Acquired Immune Deficiency Syndrome (AIDS) was first identified in the United States in June 1981 by the Centers for Disease Control and Prevention (CDC). HIV is the virus that is believed to cause AIDS and is transmitted in one of four ways: vaginal, oral or anal sex; sharing a needle for piercing, tattoos or drugs including steroids; blood products infected with HIV; and from mother to child during pregnancy, delivery or breast milk. The highest concentrations of HIV are found in the bodily fluids known to transmit HIV, blood, semen, vaginal secretions, and breast milk (Floyd, et al., 1998). Infection can occur when any of these fluids from an infected person comes into direct contact with the bloodstream or mucous membranes of another person. Trace amounts are found in tears, saliva, and other body fluids but have not been found to transmit infection. HIV is *not* spread by casual contact. It is not known if all individuals infected with this virus will develop AIDS. Women are more likely to become infected with HIV during heterosexual sex than males, because the concentration of virus is higher in semen than it is in vaginal secretions (Floyd, et al., 1998). An individual may be asymptomatic or may have some of the symptoms which include: fatigue, dry cough,

TABLE 5.1. AIDS Cases by Age	
Age	# of AIDS Cases
Under 5:	6,032
Ages 5 to 12:	1,597
Ages 13 to 19:	2,754
Ages 20 to 24:	21,097
Ages 25 to 29:	81,807
Ages 30 to 34:	133,913
Ages 35 to 39:	129,813
Ages 40 to 44:	92,986
Ages 45 to 49:	52,006
Ages 50 to 54:	27,514
Ages 55 to 59:	15,512
Ages 60 to 64:	8,716
Ages 65 or older:	7,682

Source: Centers for Disease Control and Prevention. Statistics reported to CDC through December 1996.

fever, night sweats, diarrhea, skin rashes, swollen lymph nodes, recurrent vaginal yeast infections, and/or unexplained weight loss. Typically six weeks to six months is required after the initial infection to detect the HIV antibodies in a blood test (Floyd, et al., 1998). The average time from infection until AIDS diagnosis is about ten years. There is no known cure at the present for HIV or AIDS. There are numerous drugs/cocktails (mixture of different types of drugs) that exist to boost the immune system and interfere with the replication of the virus, therefore delaying the onset of AIDS. The best way to avoid contracting HIV is to abstain from vaginal, oral or anal sex or have a mutually monogamous relationship with an uninfected partner. Other ways to protect yourself include HIV testing before becoming sexually active, consistent and correct use (See figure 5.6) of latex condoms with all sexual acts (vaginal, oral, and anal), avoid sharing needles for anything and do not have sex with anyone known or suspected of using injectable drugs including steroids.

More than 45% of those diagnosed with AIDS were infected with HIV in their teens and twenties (Floyd, et al., 1998). From 1981 to 1996, between 750,000 to 1,000,000 Americans have been diag-

TABLE 5.2. States/Territories Reporting Highest Number of AIDS Cases

State/Territory	Number of AIDS Cases
New York	106,897
California	98,157
Florida	58,911
Texas	39,871
New Jersey	32,926
Puerto Rico	18,583
Illinois	18,571
Pennsylvania	17,423
Georgia	17,004
Maryland	15,298

Metropolitan Areas Reporting Highest Number of AIDS Cases

Metropolitan Area	Number of AIDS Cases
New York City	91,799
Los Angeles	36,643
San Francisco	24,272
Miami	18,292
Washington, DC	16,787
Chicago	16,139
Houston	14,293
Philadelphia	13,325
Newark	13,213

Source: Centers for Disease Control and Prevention data as of December 1996.

nosed with HIV or AIDS. Of those, 362,000 have died from AIDS related opportunistic infections such as pneumonia (Bender, et al., 1998). Between the years of 1985 and 1994, total new diagnoses of AIDS via heterosexual contact rose from 2% to 10%, injected-drug users rose from 17% to 27%, and male homosexual contact cases fell from 67% to 44% (National Institutes of Health).

HPV

The Human Papilloma Viruses (HPV) cause warts. There are more than seventy types of HPV, several of which cause genital infections (Aral and Homes, 1991). These viruses can be transmitted by vaginal, oral or anal sex as well as skin to skin contact. Genital warts may appear three weeks to eighteen months after infection, with an average of three months (Zazove, et al., 1991). As with many of the other STIs, an individual may be infected and never show signs or symptoms of the virus. Genital warts may be brown, pink, red, yellow or grayish in color. The warts are typically found on the vaginal opening, cervix, perineum, labia, inner walls of the vagina or anal area in females and on the foreskin or shaft of the penis, anal area or urethra in males. Genital warts can cause bleeding and obstruction in the urinary and/or anal openings. There has been a strong association between HPV infection and cancers of the cervix, vagina, vulva, penis and anus (Zazove, et al., 1991; Lorincz, et al., 1992). Therefore it is imperative that all sexually active females receive an annual Pap test. It is not known if HPV directly causes cancer or if it combines with other cofactors such as infections or smoking to increase the risk of developing cancer. No cure exists at present for genital warts, however, there are treatments which decrease the size and the risk of spreading. Some of these include topical applications of podophyllin, efudex, tri-chlor, or podofilox; vaporization with a carbon dioxide laser; cauterization with an electric needle; freezing with liquid nitrogen; surgical removal; and interferon treatment (Koch, 1995). Genital/anal HPV is the most common viral STI in the United States (Aral and Holmes, 1991). Three million cases are diagnosed annually. Bauer, et al. (1991) discovered that 46 percent of female undergraduates receiving routine gynecological exams at a major California university were HPV infected.

Hepatitis B

Hepatitis B is a potentially serious and, at times, fatal illness. Currently 1,250,000 US residents are chronic carriers of Hepatitis B, of which 15 to 20% will die prematurely (4,000 to 5,500 deaths each year in the US) (Atkinson, et al., 1995). Worldwide there are 3,500,000 persons infected with Hepatitis B, which causes 1,000,000 deaths each year (Schering Corp., 1999). Fortunately, this is one of the few viruses that can be eradicated. Ninety percent of people infected with Hepatitis B eliminate the virus. This is done by developing antibodies, called immunoglobulins, which the body produces in response to the presence of the virus. These immunoglobulins (IgG and IgM) can be measured in the bloodstream and can detect whether someone has had a Hepatitis B infection. However, the remaining ten percent of individuals infected with Hepatitis B become chronic carriers. Of this group, 15–20% will die prematurely from cirrhosis or liver cancer (Schering Corp., 1999). In fact, Hepatitis B virus is second only to tobacco among the known carcinogens (Atkinson, et al., 1995). There are 140,000 to 200,000 new cases of Hepatitis B each year in the US (American Liver Foundation, 1996), with approximately 98,000 in the 15 to 39 age group (Schering Corp., 1998). One out of one hundred US residents is an infectious asymptomatic chronic carrier of Hepatitis B (Crowley, 1992). An estimated 1,250,000 Americans are currently chronic carriers, with an additional 15,000 to 20,000 new carriers per year (American Liver Foundation, 1996).

The illness is transmitted through exposure to infected blood or secretions. The disease is primarily spread through sexual contact, followed by injecting drug use (IDU). The following summarizes the routes of transmission in the US:

Heterosexual contact	41%
Homosexual contact	14%
IDU	12%
Household contacts	4%
Health care workers	2%
Unknown	25%

The concentration of Hepatitis B is high in blood and serum, and lower in semen, vaginal secretions and saliva. It can be transmitted through bites, but transmission through kissing is unlikely. There is no virus present in tears, sweat, urine or stool (Atkinson, et al., 1995). Exposure to blood from cuts, nosebleeds, menstrual bleeding and blood present on IV needles or personal items such as toothbrushes, razors and manicuring instruments may result in infection. Pregnant women pass the virus to their babies in 20 to 90% of pregnancies, dependent upon the presence or absence of certain viral components. Ninety percent of these infants become chronic carriers and twenty-five percent die of liver failure (Atkinson, et al., 1995). Other means of spreading Hepatitis B include tattooing, body piercing, sharing straws for inhaling cocaine and hemodialysis machines.

Hepatitis B is diagnosed by elevated liver enzymes (caused when liver cells are damaged and release their enzymes into the bloodstream), and the presence of Hepatitis B surface antigen (pieces of the protein coat of the virus), which is the most common test for detecting an acute infection or carrier status. Hepatitis B surface antigen can be detected as early as one to two weeks and as late as eleven to twelve weeks after exposure. If this test is positive, the person is infectious.

Once infected, the incubation period is 45–160 days, with an average of approximately 120 days. Fifty percent of adults infected are asymptomatic (Atkinson, et al., 1995). For those who are symptomatic, some or all of the following symptoms may be present. Initially (approximately two weeks after exposure) there may be diminished appetite with an approximately five to ten pound weight loss, fatigue, headache, nausea, vomiting, muscle aches, cough, low grade fever and right-sided upper abdominal pain. This is known as the 'prodrome' phase. Following the prodrome is the icteric phase, approximately one to two weeks later, which lasts two to six weeks. The urine darkens and the stools become a clay color. The liver becomes enlarged and tender. Itching is common. There may be a yellow cast to the skin or eyes. The recovery phase then follows about six to eight weeks after exposure, at which time the individual usually recovers, but may develop a chronic disease (McCance, 1994).

If a person develops a chronic disease (infection longer than six months), treatment may be necessary to diminish the risk of permanent liver damage. Interferon, which is given in these cases, is made by the body to boost immunity. The Interferon, which is used for treatment, is manufactured and given by injection for sixteen weeks to stimulate the immune system to attack the infected liver cells. The virus is completely eradicated in approximately 58% of cases (Schering Corp., 1998). However, even if there is not total elimination of the virus, the health of the liver is often improved by this treatment. New agents being currently studied are the antivirals ganciclovir and famciclovir, which appear to be promising treatments.

It is imperative that someone with chronic Hepatitis B receive the vaccine for Hepatitis A to reduce the risk of a very serious complication called acute fulminant hepatitis, in which the liver is rapidly destroyed. The death rate is 63–93% with this condition. Liver transplantation is rarely an option due to the high rate of reinfection and rapid progression of the disease after transplantation.

The CDC recommends vaccination against Hepatitis B for newborns, infants, adolescents, and those involved in high-risk behaviors, either due to occupation or lifestyle. The high cost of the vaccine prohibits universal vaccination (Benenson, 1990).

To prevent risk of exposure, one should practice 'safer sex' as detailed in the STI prevention section, avoid IV drug usage as well as sharing of toothbrushes, eating utensils, razors, nail files and clippers. If there is exposure to Hepatitis B an Immunoglobulin with a high concentration of antibody against Hepatitis B should be given within two weeks of exposure.

Parasitic STIs

Pubic Lice and Scabies

Pubic Lice (often called "crabs") and Scabies (itch mites) are tiny insects that live on the skin. They are sometimes spread sexually, but are also transmitted by contact with infected bed linens, clothes or towels (CDC.GOV). Pubic lice infect hairy parts of the body, especially around the groin area and under the arms (Tseng, 1987). With scabies, an itchy rash is the result of a female mite burrowing into a person's skin to lay her eggs. The eggs can be seen on the hair close to the skin, where they hatch in five to ten days. Some individuals infected with pubic lice have no symptoms, while others may experience considerable itching in the area infected. Light-brown insects the size of a pinhead moving on the skin or oval eggs attached to body hair may be visible (*Unspeakable.com*). The primary symptom of scabies is itching, especially at night. A rash may appear in the folds of skin between the fingers or on the wrists, elbows, abdomen or genitals (Marr, 1998). If you think you may have pubic lice or scabies, see your physician. They can determine whether treatment is necessary or not. The most effective treatments include shampoos and creams that contain lindane or a related compound. Pubic lice and scabies can be treated at home with special creams, lotions and shampoos, which are available in drugstores without a prescription. Be certain to follow the instructions carefully and do not exceed the recommended applications. The infestation may be stubborn, requiring an additional treatment. Avoid close contact with others if you have pubic lice or scabies until it is treated. Wash clothes, bed linens and any other materials that may have been infected in hot water and dry on the hottest setting. If you have pubic lice or scabies be sure to tell your sexual partner(s) or anyone with whom you have had close contact or who has shared your bed linen, clothes or towels. These individuals should be seen by a physician even if they do not have any symptoms. The best way to protect yourself is to know your partner's sexual history, don't share towels, swimsuits or underwear and thoroughly wash any materials that you think may carry pubic lice or scabies in hot water.

STI Prevention

Preventing the spread of STIs requires responsibility in sexual relationships. The best way to prevent contraction of an STI is to practice sexual abstinence or have a mutually monogamous relationship with an uninfected person and do not share needles for any reason. If an individual chooses to be sexually active, limit the number of sexual partners and use condoms consistently and correctly (See Figure 5.6). If you think you are infected, avoid any sexual contact until you visit your physician, a local STI clinic, or hospital for testing. Remember that many STIs are spread by those with no noticeable symptoms. It only takes one infected partner to contract a sexually transmitted infection.

A major problem for health care providers is persuading sexually active people to seek testing for STIs early after exposure. While some STIs such as genital herpes, HIV/AIDS and genital warts are chronic with no cure, early diagnosis can help to prevent further transmission of these infections, and in the case of herpes, early treatment of the lesions can lessen the symptoms. Symptoms of STIs can be slow to develop or may not manifest themselves at all. Thus, an individual can be infected with a number of STIs with only minor or no symptoms. For these reasons, regular and accurate evaluations are necessary to prevent the spread of STIs. Methods of testing for STIs vary with the type of infection suspected. These tests fall loosely into three categories: inspection, blood or urine testing, and/or examination of the fluids within the sores themselves or smears of fluids from the vagina or urethra. Symptomatic genital warts, herpes and pubic lice can usually be identified during an examination by a health care provider (http:\\www.unspeakable\just_the_facts, 1999). A blood test is used to test for Hepatitis B, HIV and syphilis. If the testing is done less than six months after contracting HIV and less than three weeks after contracting

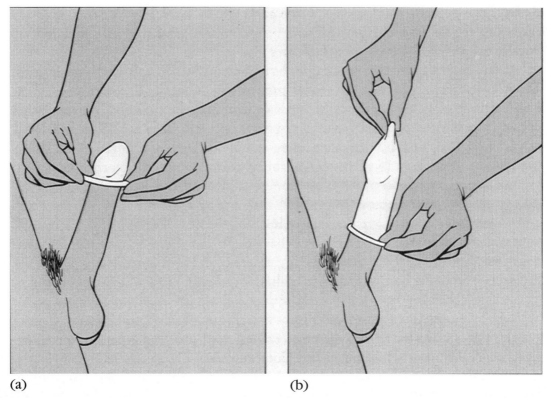

(a)   (b)

FIGURE 5.6 Using a condom. (a) The *wrong* way. (b) The *right* way: room is left at the top for the collection of semen.

From *Sexuality: Insights and Issues*, Third Edition. Copyright © 1993 by Jerrold Greenberg, Clint Buess, and Kathleen D. Mullen. Reprinted by permission of the authors.

syphilis, there is a possibility the blood test will not be sufficiently sensitive to detect the presence of the infection. A urine test for Chlamydia and gonorrhea are available at many health clinics. Often, chlamydia, gonorrhea and herpes require fluid collection from the infected site for a conclusive diagnosis (Marr, 1998). The importance of testing cannot be overemphasized. As discussed earlier, many of these infections may have dangerous complications and are easily cured. To decrease your risk of infection with an STI, you and your sexual partner(s) should know and communicate your sexual history. The only way to have adequate knowledge of your history is to be tested if there is a chance of a previous exposure regardless of the presence or absence of signs or symptoms.

Most individuals at some point in their lives will strongly desire to have children. A STI can affect the ability to conceive and have children. Chlamydia and gonorrhea can both cause males and females to become sterile. Further complications can arise for pregnant women who are in-

fected with STIs. Herpes and Hepatitis B, for example, in rare instances can be fatal to the fetus and there is a very real risk of passing HIV to a newborn. Early treatment of STIs can reduce the risk of infertility, but fertility cannot be guaranteed.

Reproduction

The *menstrual cycle* typically lasts 28 days, with a range of 20 to 40 days. Day one of the cycle is the first day of menstruation. The cycle ends with the next menstruation. (See Figure 5.7) The follicular phase begins with menstruation and terminates when ovulation occurs. The follicular phase can be very unpredictable. Stress, illness and many other factors can change when a female ovulates. This can cause problems when individuals are trying to control whether they become pregnant or not. The length of the luteal phase is much more predictable (typically 14 days), beginning with ovulation and ending when the next menstrual cycle begins (Boston Women's Health Book Collective, 1996).

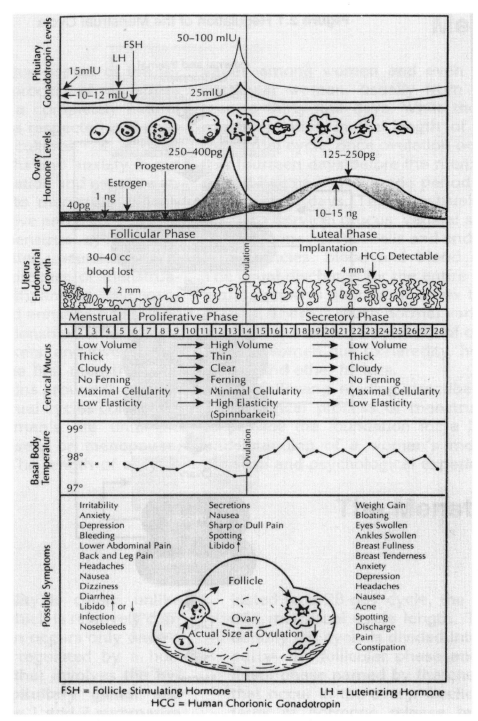

From *Contraceptive Technology,* 16th Edition by R. Hatcher. Copyright © 1994. (Irvington Publishers).

FIGURE 5.7 Menstrual Cycle Events

During the *ovarian cycle* immature eggs (follicles) are maturing and moving toward the surface of the ovary. The follicle and the ovarian surface open and allow the egg to float out. At the time of ovulation some women may feel a twinge or pain in the lower abdomen or back. After ovulation, the egg is swept into the fallopian tubes (where fertilization typically occurs) by fimbrae and the cilia (tiny hairs) and travels to the uterus. If the egg is not fertilized, it simply disintegrates or flows out with vaginal secretions, usually before menstruation. If the egg is fertilized, it will attach itself to the endometrium (internal lining of the uterus) in order to develop (Boston Women's Health Book Collective, 1996).

The *endometrial cycle* consists of three phases: the menstrual, proliferative phase and secretory phase. The menstrual phase lasts approximately four to seven days, when the lining of the uterus is sloughed off and flows out of the uterus through the vagina along with blood and other vaginal secretions. The proliferative phase lasts from the completion of the menstrual phase until ovulation. During this time the endometrium is regenerating the layer that was sloughed off with new epithelial cells. During the secretory phase the endometrium becomes twice as thick as it did during the proliferative phase. It develops a cushion-like surface, thereby possessing the ability to nourish an implanted fertilized ovum. During the end of the secretory phase, if fertilization has not occurred, the endometrium begins to deteriorate. These phases repeat throughout the reproductive years until fertilization or menopause occurs (Boston Women's Health Book Collective, 1996).

Pregnancy is usually divided into three trimesters, each of which last approximately three months or thirteen weeks (See Figure 5.8). Typically fertilization occurs 12–18 days after the beginning of the menstrual cycle. There are many variables which can impact the timing of fertilization, including irregular periods, extreme exercise, illness, stress, a missed contraceptive pill as well as many other factors. As soon as fertilization occurs the cells begin to divide and multiply. The fertilized egg implants in the uterus after approximately one

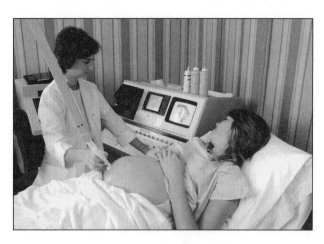

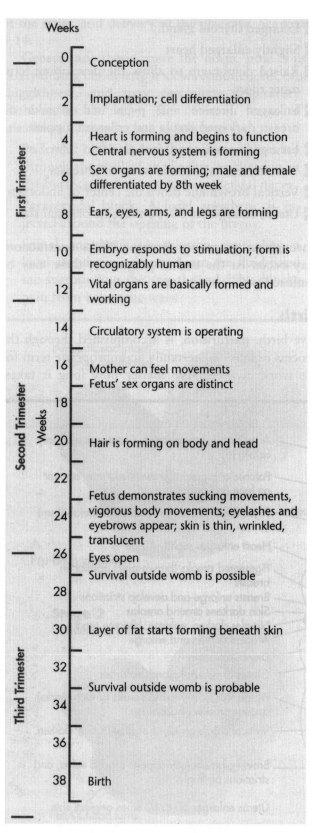

Weeks	
0	Conception
2	Implantation; cell differentiation
4	Heart is forming and begins to function Central nervous system is forming
6	Sex organs are forming; male and female differentiated by 8th week
8	Ears, eyes, arms, and legs are forming
10	Embryo responds to stimulation; form is recognizably human
12	Vital organs are basically formed and working
14	Circulatory system is operating
16	Mother can feel movements Fetus' sex organs are distinct
18	
20	Hair is forming on body and head
22	
24	Fetus demonstrates sucking movements, vigorous body movements; eyelashes and eyebrows appear; skin is thin, wrinkled, translucent
26	Eyes open Survival outside womb is possible
28	
30	Layer of fat starts forming beneath skin
32	
34	Survival outside womb is probable
36	
38	Birth

First Trimester · Second Trimester · Third Trimester

FIGURE 5.8 Prenatal development of fetus.

week. For most women the first sign(s) of pregnancy include a missed period, nausea and/or excessive fatigue. Home pregnancy kits are 97–99% accurate if used correctly. These tests can detect human chorionic gonadotropin (HCG) within two to three weeks of fertilization. HCG is the hormone secreted by the placenta to help sustain the pregnancy for the first trimester. During the second and third trimesters the HCG levels decrease and the levels of estrogen and progesterone are typically sufficient to sustain the pregnancy to term. This is believed to be the reason morning sickness ends for most women after the first trimester. The embryo develops very rapidly during the first trimester, during these three months, all of the major organs are formed. Therefore, it is imperative to see a physician as soon as an individual thinks she may be pregnant to begin taking prenatal vitamins and change any habits that could be harmful to the developing embryo. The pregnancy is dated utilizing the first day of the last menstrual period (LMP). The heartbeat can be seen during a sonogram as early as the sixth or seventh week when the embryo is approximately 5 mm long. During the second and third trimesters the fetus is growing larger and stronger in preparation for delivery. Typically the mother will begin to feel the movements of the fetus between the 16th and 20th weeks. This is referred to as "quickening". After an additional month or so, these movements can be felt externally by friends or family members. Thirty-seven weeks is considered a full term pregnancy, but typically delivery does not occur until around the 40th week.

Pregnancy Prevention

Abstinence from penile/vaginal intercourse
Effectiveness in preventing STIs and pregnancy—100%

Advantages:
- No worries
- No medical or hormonal side effects
- Protects against unwanted pregnancy

Problems:
- Very few people choose lifetime celibacy or abstinence from vaginal intercourse.
- People often forget to protect themselves against pregnancy or STIs when they stop abstaining.

Periodic Abstinence—Natural Family Planning (NFP)
Procedures:
- A woman must chart her menstrual cycle and must be able to detect certain physical signs in order to predict "unsafe" days.
- She must abstain from intercourse or use barrier contraceptives during six or more "unsafe" days each menstrual cycle.
- Check temperature daily. Before ovulation waking temperatures remain low, after ovulation temperatures rise until the next menstrual cycle begins.
- Check cervical mucus daily. Before ovulation the mucus is wet and similar to a raw egg white, after ovulation the cervical fluid dries up quickly.
- Record menstrual cycles on calendar to determine if you have regular or irregular cycles. This method is more effective for those with regular menstrual cycles.
- Remember that the sperm can live up to 72 hours after ejaculation. If a female ovulates within 72 hours after unprotected sexual intercourse the possibility of pregnancy exists.

Effectiveness in preventing pregnancy—53% to 85%; in preventing STIs—NONE

Advantages:
- No medical or hormonal side effects
- Calendars, thermometers and charts are easy to obtain

Problems:
- Taking risks during "unsafe" days
- Poor record keeping
- Illness and lack of sleep affect body temperatures
- Vaginal infections and douches change mucus
- Cannot use with irregular periods or temperature patterns

Male Condom
The latex *male condom* is a sheath, made of latex, placed over the penis prior to intercourse.

Effectiveness in preventing STIs and pregnancy—about 85%. To increase pregnancy prevention effectiveness also use spermicide or have female utilize another form of contraception.

Do not use oil-based lubricants such as Vaseline, which will cause the condom to break. Use only water based lubricants.

Advantages:
- Most effective way to prevent STIs besides abstinence
- Easy to buy (inexpensive)
- Easy to carry
- Only way for male to protect himself from unplanned pregnancy
- Can help relieve premature ejaculation

Problems:
- Possible allergies to latex
- Less sensation
- Condom breakage
- Sometimes interrupts "the mood"

The Pill

The pill (oral contraceptive pills) are a prescription medication containing the hormones estrogen and/or progestin, which prevent the release of the egg, thickens the cervical mucus and reduces the build up of the endometrial lining within the uterus. The sperm is thus unable to penetrate the egg, and/or the fertilized egg is prevented from implanting in the uterus.

Effectiveness in preventing pregnancy—97% to 99%; in preventing STIs—NONE.

Advantages:
- Nothing to put into place before intercourse
- Regular periods
- Decreases chances of developing ovarian and endometrial cancers, non-cancerous breast tumors, and ovarian cysts (Association of Reproductive Health Professionals—ARHP)
- Decreased incidence of tubal pregnancies (Planned Parenthood)

Problems:
- Must be taken daily (within the same two hour period)
- Rare but serious health risks, including: blood clots, heart attack, and stroke, which are more common for women over 35 and/or who smoke cigarettes (ARHP)
- Side effects can include temporary irregular bleeding, headaches, depression, and weight gain.

Norplant

Norplant consists of six small capsules placed under the skin which constantly release small amounts of the hormone progestin. This prevents the release of the egg, thickens the cervical mucus and reduces the build up of the endometrial lining within the uterus thereby preventing conception, and/or the fertilized egg from implanting in the uterus for five years. This procedure must be performed by a clinician and the capsules can be removed at any time. Women with the following risk factors should not use norplant: heart or liver disease, blood-clotting problems, breast cancer or smoke cigarettes.

Effectiveness in preventing pregnancy—99% (24 hours after implanted); in preventing STIs—NONE

Advantages:
- Protects against pregnancy for five years
- No daily pill
- Nothing to put in place before intercourse
- Can use while breast feeding (six weeks after delivery)
- Can be used by some women who cannot take the pill (oral contraceptive)

Problems:
- Side effects can include irregular bleeding, headaches, depression, and weight gain.
- Minor medical procedure needed for insertion and removal
- Rarely, infection at insertion site
- Expensive

Depo-Provera

Depo-Provera is a hormone shot injected into the arm or buttocks every 12 weeks, which will prevent the release of the egg, thickens the cervical mucus and reduces the build up of the endometrial lining within the uterus thereby preventing conception, and/or the fertilized egg from implanting in the uterus.

Effectiveness in preventing pregnancy—99%; in preventing STIs—NONE

Advantages:
- Protects against pregnancy for 12 weeks
- No daily pill
- Nothing to put in place before intercourse
- Can be used by some women who cannot take the pill (oral contraceptive)
- Decreases incidence of cancer in the lining of the uterus as well as iron deficiency anemia (ARHP)
- Provides privacy—no pill pack

Problems:
- Side effects include irregular bleeding, headaches, depression, abdominal pains and often no periods at all
- Side effects cannot be reversed until medication wears off (up to 12 weeks)
- May cause delay in getting pregnant after shots are stopped (up to 12—18 months)

Diaphragm and Cervical Cap

Latex cup (diaphragm) or thimble shaped (cervical cap) require fitting by a clinician. The diaphragm or cap is coated with spermicide before placement in the vagina. The diaphragm or cervical cap combined with spermicide act by destroying the sperm and preventing the sperm from reaching the egg.

Effectiveness in preventing pregnancy—Diaphragm with spermicide—82% to 94%; Cervical cap with spermicide—82%; in preventing STIs—NONE

Advantages:
- No major health concerns
- Can last several years

Problems:
- More difficult preparation
- Possibility of allergies to latex or spermicide
- Cannot use with vaginal bleeding or an infection
- Diaphragm—increased risk of bladder infection
- Cervical Cap—difficult for some women to use and/or difficult to fit some women

- Refitting is necessary with a gain or loss of more than 10 pounds

Over the Counter Contraceptives for Women

Procedures:

Female condom—insert vaginal pouch prior to intercourse

Spermicide, foam, jelly or cream—insert into vagina prior to intercourse

Effectiveness in preventing pregnancy—Female condom—74% to 79%

Spermicide, foam, jelly or cream—70% to 80%

Female condom in preventing STIs—similar to the male condom, but not quite as effective, due to possible folding.
Spermicides, foam, jelly and cream in preventing STIs—NONE

Advantages:
- Easy to purchase in drugstores, supermarkets, etc.
- Increased sensation compared to the male condom

Problems:
- Expensive (female condom)
- Outer ring of female condom may slip into vagina during intercourse
- Possible difficulty inserting the pouch
- More difficult preparation
- Possible allergies to spermicide

IUD

The intrauterine device (IUD) requires a health care professional to insert a small plastic device into the uterus. The IUD contains copper or hormones which impede conception or prevent implantation of a fertilized egg.

Effectiveness in preventing pregnancy—95% to 96%; in preventing STIs—NONE

Advantages:
- Nothing to put into place before intercourse
- Copper IUD may be left in place for up to eight years
- No daily pills

TABLE 5.3 Prevention of Sexually Transmitted Infections (STIs) and Pregnancy

Birth Control Method	Effectiveness in Preventing Pregnancy	Effectiveness in Preventing Sexually Transmitted Infections
Abstinence from Penile/Vaginal Intercourse	100%	100%
Periodic Abstinence	53% to 85%	0%
Male Condom	Approximately 85%	Approximately 85%
Oral Contraceptive Pill	97% to 99%	0%
Norplant Implant	99%	0%
Depo-Provera Injection	99%	0%
Diaphragm/Cervical Cap	82% to 94%	0%
Female Condom	74% to 79%	74% to 79%
Intrauterine Device	95% to 96%	0%
Sterilization	99%	0%

(Floyd, et al., 1998)

Problems:

- May cause cramping
- Spotting between periods
- Heavier and longer periods
- Increased risk of tubal infection, which may lead to sterility (Planned Parenthood)
- Rarely, the wall of the uterus is punctured (Floyd et al., 1998)
- Not recommended for anyone who has never had a child
- Not recommended for anyone not in a mutually monogamous relationship

Sterilization

Sterilization is an operation performed on the female (tubal ligation) or male (vasectomy).

Procedures:

The *tubal ligation* is intended to permanently block a woman's fallopian tubes, where sperm typically unite with the egg.

A *vasectomy* is preformed to permanently block a man's vas deferens tubes, which transport sperm.

Effectiveness in preventing pregnancy—99%; in preventing STIs—NONE

Advantages:

- Permanent protection against pregnancy
- No lasting side effects
- No effects on sexual pleasure
- Protects woman whose health would be seriously threatened by a pregnancy

Problems:

- Mild bleeding or infection after the surgery
- Some people eventually regret being unable to have children later in life
- Reaction to anesthetic
- Reversibility cannot be guaranteed
- Rarely, tubes reopen, allowing pregnancy to occur
- Rare complications with tubal ligation include bleeding and injury to the bowel
- Vasectomy—infection or blood clot can occur in or near the testicles; often there is temporary bruising, swelling, or tenderness of the scrotum

Emergency Contraception

After unprotected intercourse, emergency contraception may be utilized. This treatment has been in place for several years in other countries, but only recently became available in the U.S. The medication should be taken within 72 hours of unprotected sexual intercourse and is typically used in rape or broken condom situations. This is effective 75% of the time, with pregnancy resulting in 25% of the cases. Some common side effects include significant nausea and vomiting. This is not to be used as a regular method of birth control. As with many of the other pregnancy prevention methods, this

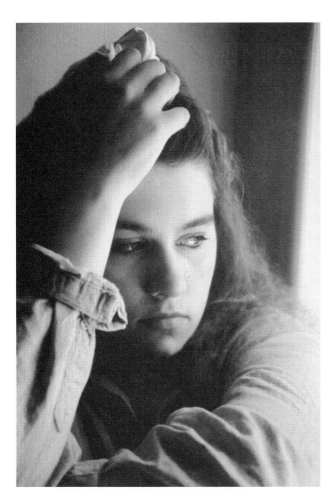

pen, while for others parenthood is quite difficult and challenging. For most, this phase of life (given its rewards and demands) is a blend of these two perspectives. These differences of opinion are often influenced by the stage of life during which the individual becomes a parent, combined with factors such as other life circumstances (whether the parent will be a single parent or not) as well as the personality and financial situation of the new parent. Parenthood usually will dramatically alter the lifestyle to which an individual has become accustomed. Initially, it is an end to restful nights, spur of the moment trips, and many social activities. New parents now have an individual who is solely dependent upon them 24 hours a day for attention, love, food, clothing, safety and shelter. This can be overwhelming physically, mentally and financially even for the most prepared parents. It is also a time of tremendous joy as well as many special moments, such as your baby's first smile, giggle, word or step. As the child grows they are less dependent upon you for the basic necessities but those needs change into dance lessons, soccer practice and

one offers no protection against the contraction of STIs.

Unplanned Pregnancy

This can be a very exciting and/or frightening time in an individual's life. The thought of pregnancy conjures up many emotions, such as the realization of life changes, increased responsibility, happiness and worry all at the same time. Pregnancy and the responsibilities of parenthood are tremendous. It is important to realize these potential consequences of unprotected intercourse or failed pregnancy prevention exist. It is a good idea to discuss how you might handle this situation with your *potential* sexual partner. In the event of an unplanned pregnancy, there are several options, none of which are easy and all can be life altering. These will be discussed in the following sections.

Parenthood

Parenthood has been described in many words. Many agree it is one of the best things that can hap-

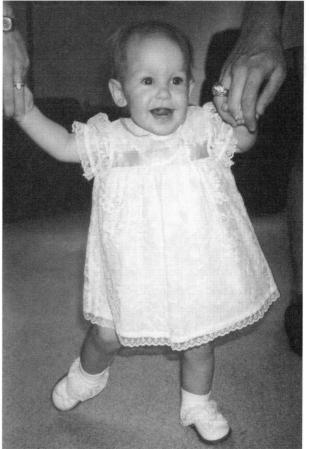

slumber parties, to name a few. The commitment to becoming a parent is large and one that never ends and can be very difficult to face alone.

Adoption

For many, present life circumstances do not permit them to remain the caregiver in the best interest of their child. Many factors, such as the age of the parent and economic circumstance, come to bear upon this complex and often difficult decision. For the vast majority this is indeed a most difficult decision to reach. The bond that ties the newborn child and parent(s) is enormous. Usually this course is taken in an attempt to be unselfish and provide the child with improved opportunities in life which might otherwise be unavailable to them. Many adoption agencies exist to help make this option as painless as possible. There are many different types of adoptions. Some allow the biological parents to remain a part of the child's life; others do not, but provide a mechanism whereby the child can eventually obtain information regarding the biological parents. Often this information can be made available only after the adopted child enters adolescence or adulthood. Sometimes people believe adoption will make their problems go away, this is often not the case. Some experience regrets about putting a child up for adoption years later and are plagued with "what ifs".

Abortion

Some individuals cannot (due to medical reasons) or do not want to carry the embryo to term, and therefore choose abortion. This decision is reached for various reasons. Sometimes this is felt to be the best decision because of the circumstances of conception (such as a rape resulting in pregnancy). Some believe they cannot disclose a pregnancy to their parents or partner and see no other alternative. Others are not ready to become parents and do not want to complete the pregnancy. Many people believe that if the pregnancy is terminated their problems will disappear, but this is often not the case. Some experience regrets years after an abortion and are plagued with "what ifs".

As mentioned earlier, pregnancy is accompanied by many emotions and lasting effects for both partners. There is no easy route once pregnancy has occurred. It is a good idea to discuss your values and ideas of what you would do in the event of

an unplanned pregnancy with your prospective sexual partner. It is best to fully consider all of the options before making a decision.

References

Aral, S., & Holmes, K. 1991. Sexually Transmitted Diseases in the AIDS Era. *Scientific American,* 264: 62–69.

Association of Reproductive Health Professionals. ARHP.

Bauer, H., et al. 1991. Genital Human Papillomavirus Infection in Female University Students as Determined by a PCR-based Method. *Journal of the American Medical Association,* 265: 472–477.

Bender, D., et al. *AIDS: Opposing Viewpoints.* San Diego, CA: Greenhaven Press 1998.

Boston Women's Health Book Collective. *The New Our Bodies, Ourselves.* 25th anniversary ed. New York, NY: Touchstone 1996.

Center for Disease Control. 1996.

Center for Prevention Services U.S. Venereal Disease Control Division. Documents Div/U.S. Docs Dept. Washington, DC.

Crowley, L. *Introduction to Human Disease.* 3rd ed. Boston, MA: Jones and Bartlett Publishers, Inc 1992.

Crum, C., and Ellner, P. (1985). "Chlamydial Infections: Making the diagnosis." *Contemporary Obstetrics and Gynecology,* 25, 153–159, 163, 165, 168.

Floyd, P., et al. *Personal Health: Perspectives & Lifestyles* (2nd ed.). (Englewood, CO: Morton Publishing Co 1998)

Kassler, W., and Cates, W. (1992). "The Epidemiology and Prevention of Sexually Transmitted Diseases." *Urological Clinics of North America,* 19, 1–12.

Keim, J., et al. (1992). "Screening for Chlamydia Trachomatis in College Women on Routine Gynecological Exams." *Journal of American College Health,* 41, 17–23.

Koch, P. *Exploring Our Sexuality: An Interactive Text* (Preliminary ed.). (Dubuque, IA: Kendall/Hunt Publishing Co 1995)

Lee, H. (1989). "Genital Chlamydial Infection in Female and Male College Students." *Journal of American College Health,* 37, 288–291.

Lorincz, A., et al. (1992). "Human Papillomavirus Infection of the Cervix: Relative Risk Associa-

tion of 15 Common Anogenital Types."
Obstetrics and Gynecology, 79, 328–337.

Marr, L. *Sexually Transmitted Diseases: A Physician Tells You What You Need to Know.* (Baltimore, MD: John Hopkins University Press 1998)

Microsoft Encarta (1997).

Moglia, R., and Knowles, J. (eds) *All about Sex.* (New York, NY: Three Rivers Press 1997)

National Institutes of Health. (From AIDS Opposing Viewpoints, pg. 30)

Planned Parenthood.

Sloane, E. *Biology of Women* (3rd ed.). (Albany, NY: Delmar Publishers 1993)

Strong, B., et al. *Core Concepts in Human Sexuality.* (Mountain View, CA: Mayfield Publishing Co 1996)

Tseng, C. *Sexually Transmitted Diseases: A Handbook of Protection, Prevention, and Treatment.* (Saratonga, CA: R&E Publishers 1987)

http:\\www.unspeakable\just_the_facts, 1999

Zazove, P., et al. (1991). "Genital Human Papillomavirus Infection." *American Family Physician,* 43, 1279–1291.

Contacts

Aggie Health Ring
http://health.tamu.edu/

AIDS Treatment Information Service
800-HIV-0440
http://www.hivatis.org

AIDS Services of Brazos Valley
1702-B South Texas Avenue, Suite 202
Bryan, TX 77802
979-260-2437
http://www.aids@myriad.net

Brazos County Health Department
201 North Texas Avenue
Bryan, TX 77803
979-361-4440

BVCAA Family Planning Clinic
3400 S. Texas Ave., Suite 1
Bryan, TX 77802
979-268-5555 ext. 3

CDC National STI Hotline
800-227-8922
http://www.sunsite.unc.edu/ASHA/

CDC National AIDS Hotline
800-342-AIDS(2437)
http://sunsite.unc.edu/ASHA/

Center for Disease Control
http://www.cdc.gov

Emergency Contraception Hotline
800-584-9911

Gender Issues Education Services
979-845-1107
http://stulife.tamu.edu/gies/

Gladney Center for Adoption
713-665-1212

Good Samaritan Pregnancy Services
505 University Drive E
Bryan, TX 77802
979-846-2909

Healthfinder
http://www.healthfinder.gov

Herpes Resource Center
800-230-6039
http://sunsite.unc.edu/ASHA/herpes/hrc.html

Hope Pregnancy Centers of Brazos County
3620 East 29th
Bryan, TX 77802
979-846-1097

http://www.unspeakable.com/facts

Info Tex 979-268-0378
(Enter any 4-digit code below when prompted.)
    7143 AIDS
    7144 Gonorrhea
    7145 Herpes
    7146 Syphilis

International Childbirth Education Association
612-854-8660
http://www.ICEA.org

JAMA HIV/AIDS Information Center
www.ama-assn.org/special/hiv/

National Abortion Federation
800-772-9100
http://www.cais.com/naf

National Council on Adoption
202-328-1200
http://www.ncfa-usa.org

National Herpes Hotline
800-230-6039
http://www.unspeakable.com/facts

North American Council on Adoptable Children
    (NACAC)
612-644-3036
http://www.cyfc.umn.edu/adoptinfo/NACAC.html

Planned Parenthood
4112 East 29th
Bryan, TX 77802
979-846-1744
http://www.plannedparenthood.org

Project Rachel
888-456-4673

Shanti Project
(Counseling and assistance for persons with AIDS)
415-864-2273
http://www.shanti.org

Texas A&M University Health Center
979-845-1511
http://shs.tamu.edu/
979-847-8910
http://healthed.tamu.edu/

Activities

In-Class Activities

Apply % incidence of STIs, HIV, unplanned pregnancy, adoption and abortion to class size.

The "Perfect" Mate

Where Do You Rank?

Can We Make Ends Meet?

Passive Listening

Active Listening

Compromise

Notebook Activities

What Is Your Risk of Contracting a Sexually Transmitted Infection?

STD Risk Profiler (www.unspeakable.com/nph-survey.cgi?tag=risk)

STD Quiz (www.unspeakable.com/nph-survey.cgi?tag=std)

STI Attitudes

Successful Contraception Questionnaire (www.arhp.org/success/index.html)

■ The "Perfect" Mate (RC-22)

Directions: In the space below, write down all the qualities of a "perfect" mate for you. Then go back over the list and write the codes that apply in the blank to the left.

Qualities of my "Perfect" Mate:

_____ 1.

_____ 2.

_____ 3.

_____ 4.

_____ 5.

_____ 6.

_____ 7.

_____ 8.

_____ 9.

_____ 10.

_____ 11.

_____ 12.

_____ 13.

_____ 14.

_____ 15.

_____ 16.

_____ 17.

_____ 18.

_____ 19.

_____ 20.

Codes:

D   Your dad has this quality.

M   Your mom has this quality.

+   You have this quality.

–   You wish you had this quality.

B   You think both partners need this quality to be happy.

*   These are the three most important qualities.

■ Where Do You Rank? (RC-23)

Directions: Rank each statement from 1 to 3 with one being the best choice and 3 being the worst choice.

1. Which would be hardest for you to accept?

   _____ Your husband or wife cheating on you.

   _____ Your husband or wife becoming dependent on "hard" drugs.

   _____ Finding out your husband or wife was married before, but never told you.

2. What do you look for in a mate?

   _____ someone who is good-looking

   _____ someone who has a lot of money

   _____ someone who is fun to be with

3. What do you look at first when you see someone of the opposite sex?

   _____ their eyes

   _____ their overall figure

   _____ their face

4. Which one of these would you most want to avoid in a relationship?

   _____ boredom

   _____ no communication

   _____ little intimacy

5. Which of these is most preferable to you?

   _____ staying single

   _____ getting married but no kids

   _____ getting married and having kids

6. How would you prefer to meet someone?

   _____ in class

   _____ on a blind date

   _____ at the mall

7. Which best describes you?

   _____ don't like public displays of affection

   _____ hugging is OK in public

   _____ hugging and kissing are OK in public

■ Activity 10: Can We Make Ends Meet?

Concept/
Description: Being a parent can drastically change a person's life socially, emotionally, physically, and financially.

Objective: To explore the financial strain that being a parent would cause the typical college student.

Materials: Classified section of the newspaper
Parents sheet (RC-28)
Parents (2) sheet (RC-29)
Pens or pencils

Directions:
1. Divide the class into groups of four and give each group the Parents sheets.
2. Ask each group to choose a job from the classified section for which the would be qualified. Assuming that they got the job, estimate how much money they would make in a year. (Call the company, if possible.)
3. Give students a few days to research the information on the sheets by asking people, calling various companies to get rates, etc.
4. Fill in the sheets and figure out if your "income" could cover your "expenses."
5. Ask students to list the many difficulties parents face, besides financial strain.
6. Discuss.

■ Parents (RC-28)

Directions: Being a parent can drastically change your life. Figure out the financial aspect of being a parent by filling in the information below:

HOUSING

1. Rent $ _____ per month

2. Utilities

    Gas $ _____ per month
    Electricity $ _____ per month
    Garbage $ _____ per month
    Water $ _____ per month
    Sewer $ _____ per month

3. Approximate phone bill $ _____ per month

4. Cable television $ _____ per month

    TOTAL $ _____ PER MONTH

AUTO

1. Car payment $ _____ per month

2. Gasoline $ _____ per month

3. Car repairs $ _____ per month

4. License and insurance $ _____ per month

    TOTAL $ _____ PER MONTH

BABY

1. Day care $ _____ per month

2. Diapers $ _____ per month

3. Baby clothing $ _____ per month

    TOTAL $ _____ PER MONTH

■ Parents (2) (RC-29)

G E N E R A L

1. Food bill $ _____ per month

2. Health care $ _____ per month

3. Entertainment $ _____ per month

4. Savings $ _____ per month

5. Miscellaneous (gifts, toys, etc.)

                              TOTAL $ _____ PER MONTH

TOTALS:

Housing	$ _____	_____
Auto	$ _____	_____
Baby	$ _____	_____
General	$ _____	_____
TOTAL MONTHLY COSTS	$ _____	_____

Do you think that a typical college student could make ends meet?
Why or why not?

■ Passive Listening (RC-42)

Directions: Passive listening is showing a person that you are interested without really speaking. In the box below, you will find some passive listening techniques. Choose one of the topics for discussion from the Topics for Discussion sheet (RC-44) and, with a partner, have a conversation with one person speaking and the other listening passively. Change roles so that both will get a chance to speak and listen. When finished, answer the questions below the box.

Passive Listening Techniques

Make eye contact.
Nod your head.
Lean forward.
Reflect your feelings with facial expressions.
Use short encouraging verbal responses ("uh-huh").

---

1. When you were the listener, did you find it difficult to remain quiet? Why or why not?

2. Did you have to concentrate on listening passively or did it come naturally?

3. Have you ever spoken to someone who couldn't wait to voice his or her opinion? How could you tell? Describe his or her body language.

4. Did you like speaking with a passive listener? Why or why not?

5. Did your partner appear interested in what you were saying? How did that make y ou feel?

■ Active Listening (RC-43)

Directions: Active listening is using verbal responses to show acceptance, understanding, respect, sympathy, and encouragement. In the box are some active listening techniques. Choose one of hte topics for discussion from the Topics for Discussion sheet (RC-44) and, with a partner, have a conversation with one person speaking and the other listening actively. Change roles so that both will get a chance to speak and listen. When finished, answer the questions below the box.

Active Listening Techniques

Use verbal responses ("Really?," "I see," "What happened next?").
Comment directly on what is being said.
Restate the speaker's ideas in your own words ("Do you mean...?").
Encourage the person to express feelings ("I guess you must have felt...").
Encourage more information ("Tell me about...").
Don't pass judgment.

---

1. When you were the listener, did you find it difficult to use active listening? Why or why not?

2. Did you have to concentrate on active listening or did it come naturally?

3. Have you ever spoken to someone who constantly interrupted you? How did that make you feel?

4. Did you like speaking with an active listener? Why or why not?

5. Did your partner appear genuinely interested in what you were saying or were you aware that he or she was trying to use active listening? Explain.

■ Topics for Discussion (RC-44)

1. Describe one of the funniest situations you have ever been in.

2. Tell about the scariest thing that ever happened to you.

3. Tell about the proudest moment in your life.

4. Talk about someone you admire and why.

5. Talk about your favorite actor or actress and why you like him or her.

6. In your opinion, what was the greatest moment in sports?

7. Talk about your best moment in sports.

8. What is your greatest accomplishment?

9. What talents to you possess? Explain.

10. Talk about your favorite vacation.

11. What is the worst time you've ever had on a vacation.

12. If someone gave you $100,000, what would you do with it?

13. What is your greatest fear? Explain.

14. If you could go anywhere in the world, where would you go and why?

15. If you could change one thing about the world, what would you change and why?

■ Compromise (RC-54)

Directions: Compromising is giving up something in order to reach an agreement. It is a process of giving and taking to agree on a common goal. Using the situations listed, first brainstorm the solutions, then compromise on the final decision. The guidelines for compromising are listed below:

Compromise Guidelines:

1. Everyone *must* get a chance to voice an opinion.
2. All group members have a say in the final decision.
3. Any decision must be approved by *everyone* in the group.
4. *Everyone* must agree to support the final decision.

Compromise Topics

1. If you could invite any famous person to your school for one day, who should be invited?

2. A gift of $200,000 was given to your school by a wealthy graduate. How should the money be spent?

3. The school has decided to give your group an all-expense paid trip to anywhere in the world for one week. Where will you go?

■ STD Risk Profiler

http://www.unspeakable.com/nph-survey.cgi?tag=risk

Are you male or female?	☐ Male	☐ Female
What age group are you in ?	☐ -25	☐ 25-40 ☐ 40+
Do you live in a city of more than 200,000?	☐ Yes	☐ No
Have you had sex with more than one partner in the past three months?	☐ Yes	☐ No
Have you had sex with a new partner in the past three months?	☐ Yes	☐ No
Do you know or suspect that your partner has had sex with other partners?	☐ Yes	☐ No
Have you ever had sex without using a condom?	☐ Yes	☐ No
Have you ever had sex with someone the first time you met?	☐ Yes	☐ No
Have you ever had an STD?	☐ Yes	☐ No
Have you ever had sex after using drugs or alcohol?	☐ Yes	☐ No
Have you or your partner ever used cocaine?	☐ Yes	☐ No
Have you or your partner ever used IV drugs?	☐ Yes	☐ No
Have you ever given someone money or drugs in exchange for sex?	☐ Yes	☐ No

■ STD Quiz

http://www.unspeakable.com/nph-survey.cgi?tag=std

Few of us know as much as we should about sexually transmitted diseases (STDs). Take this opportunity to test your knowledge of STDs, and learn more about their symptoms, prevention, and treatment. Submit your answers to find out the naked truth.

Note: The STD Quiz is an anonymous service provided to you solely for educational purposes. Absolutely no information about you is collected by this program. You are the only person who can view the results, which are discarded forever when your browser session ends.

1. 40 million Americans currently have:
   - ☐ a) HIV/AIDS
   - ☐ b) herpes
   - ☐ c) chlamydia

2. Women who've had an STD are at increased risk for:
   - ☐ a) infertility
   - ☐ b) HIV/AIDS
   - ☐ c) cervical cancer

3. Which of the following bacterial STDs do experts call "the silent epidemic"?
   - ☐ a) scabies
   - ☐ b) chlamydia
   - ☐ c) trichomoniasis

4. Which of the following groups is at greatest risk for STDs?
   - ☐ a) men under 25
   - ☐ b) women under 25
   - ☐ c) men 25-40

5. When asked to name the greatest obstacle they face in trying to protect themselves against STDs, people most often cite:
   - ☐ a) carelessness
   - ☐ b) ignorance
   - ☐ c) self-consciousness

6. Experts now recommend that sexually active young people be immunized against what STD?
   - ☐ a) chlamydia
   - ☐ b) herpes
   - ☐ c) hepatitis B

7. Which of the following STDs can be cured?
   - ☐ a) herpes
   - ☐ b) gonorrhea
   - ☐ c) genital warts

8. For women, the most common symptom of chlamydia and gonorrhea infection is:
   ☐ a) vaginal discharge
   ☐ b) sores and/or blisters in the genital region
   ☐ c) no symptom

9. You may be at increased risk for HIV/AIDS if:
   ☐ a) you have had many sex partners in the last 10 years
   ☐ b) you have given blood at a blood bank or blood collection center
   ☐ c) you have eaten food prepared by a person infected with HIV

10. The best form of protection against contracting STDs during sex is:
    ☐ a) spermicides
    ☐ b) condoms, used correctly all the time
    ☐ c) birth control pills

■ STI Attitudes

Directions: Please read each statement carefully. STI means sexually transmissible infection. Record your reaction by circling the number.

Use This Key: 1 = Strongly Agree   2 = Agree   3 = Undecided   4 = Disagree   5 = Strongly Disagree

1 2 3 4 5   1. How one uses one's sexuality has nothing to do with getting an STI.

1 2 3 4 5   2. It is easy to use the prevention methods that reduce one's chances of getting an STI.

1 2 3 4 5   3. Responsible sex is one of the best ways of reducing the risk of STIs.

1 2 3 4 5   4. Getting early medical care is the main key to preventing harmful effects of STIs.

1 2 3 4 5   5. Choosing the right sex partner is important in reducing the risk of getting an STI.

1 2 3 4 5   6. A high rate of STI should be a concern for all people.

1 2 3 4 5   7. People with an STI have a duty to get their sex partners to medical care.

1 2 3 4 5   8. The best way to get a sex partner to STI treatment is to take him/her to the doctor with you.

1 2 3 4 5   9. Changing one's sex habits is necessary once the presence of an STI is known.

1 2 3 4 5   10. I would dislike having to follow the medical steps for treating an STI.

1 2 3 4 5   11. If I were sexually active, I would feel uneasy doing things before and after sex to prevent getting an STI.

1 2 3 4 5   12. If I were sexually active, it would be insulting if a sex partner suggested we use a condom to avoid STI.

1 2 3 4 5   13. I dislike talking about STIs with my peers.

1 2 3 4 5   14. I would be uncertain about going to the doctor unless I was sure I really had an STI.

1 2 3 4 5   15. I would feel that I should take my sex partner with me to a clinic if I thought I had an STI.

1 2 3 4 5   16. It would be embarrassing to discuss STI with one's partner if one were sexually active.

1 2 3 4 5   17. If I were to have sex, the chance of getting an STI makes me uneasy about having sex with more than one person.

1 2 3 4 5   18. I like the idea of sexual abstinence (not having sex) as the best way of avoiding STIs.

1 2 3 4 5   19. If I had an STI, I would cooperate with public health people to find the source of STIs.

1 2 3 4 5   20. If I had an STI, I would avoid exposing others while I was being treated.

1 2 3 4 5   21. I would have regular STI checkups if I were having sex with more than one partner.

1 2 3 4 5   22. I intend to look for STI signs before deciding to have sex with anyone.

1 2 3 4 5   23. I will limit my sex activity to just one partner because of the chances I might get an STI.

1 2 3 4 5   24. I will avoid sex contact anytime I think there is even a slight chance of getting an STI.

1 2 3 4 5   25. The chance of getting an STI would not stop me from having sex.

1 2 3 4 5   26. If I had a chance, I would support community efforts toward controlling STIs.

1 2 3 4 5   27. I would be willing to work with others to make people aware of STI problems in my town.

Calculate your total points using the following point values. For items 1, 10–14, 16, and 25: reverse the scoring of your circled response (1 becomes 5, 2 becomes 4, and so on). For Items 2–9, 15, 17–24, 26, and 27: add the points as you have them circled. The higher your score, the stronger your predisposition to engage in high-risk STI behaviors. The lower your score, the stronger your predisposition to practice low-risk STI behaviors. The range for the score is 27–135.

■ Successful Contraception
http://www.arhp.org/success/index.html

Choose with Care. Use with Confidence.

Answer the questions below. Remember, there are no right or wrong answers. The exercise should take you no more than 15 minutes to complete. When you finish the survey, *you'll get a profile of birth control options that appear best suited for you, based on your medical history and your lifestyle.* This questionnaire is limited to the most popular and effective contraceptive groups which are:

> oral contraceptives ("the pill")
> prescription barrier methods ("diaphragms and cervical caps")
> non-prescription barrier methods ("condoms and spermicides")
> intrauterine device ("IUD")
> implants ("Norplant")
> injectables ("Depo-Provera")
> sterilization

Each of these contraceptives has been proven highly effective and safe if used properly. The questionnaire does not address abstinence or early withdrawal. Keep in mind that using a combination of a latex or polyurethane condom and other methods can help protect you against both pregnancy and diseases, like AIDS, that are transmitted through sexual contact.

While some contraceptives have side effects, these can often be handled effectively. Some methods, such as the pill, also offer many health benefits. The key to successful contraception is getting to know your birth control method. Ask questions of your health care provider and others, and discuss your choices with your partner.

General Questions

- Are you male or female?　　　☐ Female　　☐ Male
  (If Male, please note: Contraception options available for men include *condoms* and *sterilization*. To find out more about these options, please click on the option you would like to learn more about.)
- Are you under age 35?　　　☐ Under 35　　☐ Over 35
- Have you had any children?　　　☐ Yes　☐ No
- Are you pregnant now?　　　☐ Yes　☐ No

Questions about Lifestyle Choices

The next set of questions looks at some of the lifestyle choices you make and how they can affect your birth control options. Your profile of options should only include methods that you know you will be comfortable using...and methods that match the pattern of your sex life.

- Do you have more than one sex partner?　　☐ Yes　☐ No
- How often do you have sexual intercourse?　　☐ Frequently　☐ Not frequently
- Do you ever have sex with a partner who you suspect may be at risk of being exposed to HIV (the AIDS virus)?　　☐ Yes　☐ No
- If a birth control method, such as a diaphragm, cervical cap or condom, interrupts lovemaking, will you prefer not using it?　　☐ Yes　☐ No
- On a scale of 1 to 5 where 1 means you hate routines and 5 means you function best when you have a set routine, where would you place yourself?　　☐ 1　☐ 2　☐ 3　☐ 4　☐ 5

Reprinted by permission of the Association of Reproductive Professionals.

- In general, does learning that a contraceptive contains hormones make you more likely or less likely to use it, or does it make no difference?　　☐ More　　☐ Less　　☐ No Difference

Health Matters Questions

When choosing a birth control method, it is understandable that you will want to know the method's risks. The good news is most forms of birth control are extremely safe for many women. However, some birth control methods may not be appropriate for you because of your health.

Most of the health problems that prevent you from safely using a birth control method are relatively rare, especially in young women. If you think you may have any of the medical conditions in the 'Medical History' section below, you should consult with your health care provider. And remember that answering the following questions does not take the place of a discussion with your health care provider about which birth control method is right for you.

- Do you smoke?　　☐ Yes　　☐ No
- Do you have difficulty with shots?　　☐ Yes　　☐ No
- Do you plan to get pregnant within the next five years?　　☐ Yes　　☐ No
- Do you plan to get pregnant within the next 12 months?　　☐ Yes　　☐ No
- Do you want the choice of ever getting pregnant?　　☐ Yes　　☐ No
- Do you have ready access to a health care provider?　　☐ Yes　　☐ No

Questions About Your Medical History

Because some medical conditions may make certain contraceptive methods inappropriate for you, your health care provider will probably ask you questions regarding your medical history. Be sure to consult with your health care provider when deciding which method is best for you.

To further refine your contraceptive options, please answer "yes" or "no" to the following medical history questions:

Have you ever been told by a health care provider that you have any of the following medical conditions:

Blood clots	Diabetes	Frequent fainting
☐ Yes　☐ No	☐ Yes　☐ No	☐ Yes　☐ No
Active cervical infection	Gall bladder disease	Severe anemia
☐ Yes　☐ No	☐ Yes　☐ No	☐ Yes　☐ No
Impaired liver function or liver tumors	Abnormal pap smear that has not been resolved	Pregnancy in the past six weeks
☐ Yes　☐ No	☐ Yes　☐ No	☐ Yes　☐ No
Known or suspected breast cancer	Severe headaches, particularly migraines	Heavy menstrual bleeding or cramping
☐ Yes　☐ No	☐ Yes　☐ No	☐ Yes　☐ No
Abnormal vaginal bleeding	Pelvic infection (PID)	Uterine fibroid tumors
☐ Yes　☐ No	☐ Yes　☐ No	☐ Yes　☐ No
High blood pressure	Ectopic pregnancy	Depression
☐ Yes　☐ No	☐ Yes　☐ No	☐ Yes　☐ No
Pelvic or abdominal surgery		
☐ Yes　☐ No		

Questionnaire is complete.

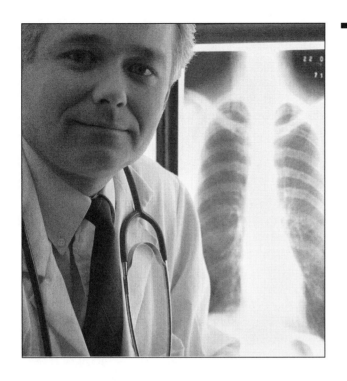

Chapter Six

Diseases

"Habits are to the soul what the veins and arteries are to the blood, the courses in which it moves."

—Horace Bushnell

OBJECTIVES

Students will be able to:

• differentiate between communicable and non-communicable diseases

• identify the symptoms of various diseases

• list five strategies which should be utilized by members of their age group to avoid contraction of these diseases

• know the risk factors for cancer

• identify the seven warning signs of cancer

• be able to list the steps for the breast self-exam (BSE) and testicular self-exam (TSE)

• list important aspects of periodic self/doctor examinations

• differentiate between Type I and Type II diabetes

• list three risk factors for type II diabetes

• define and describe anemia

• know the signs and symptoms of anemia

• identify three possible causes of ulcers

The purpose of this chapter is to inform individuals regarding symptoms, methods of transmission, precautions and treatments of communicable and non-communicable diseases most common to the college aged population.

Communicable Diseases

Communicable diseases are those diseases that are transmitted from person to person. These diseases can be transmitted directly by physical contact, which can include coughing or sneezing or indirectly by contaminated water or infected insects.

HIV/AIDS (Non-Sexual Contraction)

Can be contracted through blood transfusions, sharing needles, and/or the exchange of blood or breast milk from a mother to her unborn or newborn child. The groups that have been found to be at higher risk include IV drug users and those individuals who received a blood transfusion before 1985.

Tuberculosis

Tuberculosis (TB) is a communicable disease which primarily affects the lungs and was responsible for a large number of deaths and disabilities until the middle of this century. There was a sharp decline in the devastation caused by this illness from 1950 to

1980 due to the discovery of effective medications. However there has been an increase of approximately 16% in the incidence of TB during the past decade as a result of a number of factors which will be discussed later.

Tuberculosis is caused primarily by the bacillus (or rod-shaped) microorganism Mycobacterium tuberculosis; other Mycobacteria strains are responsible for some cases, particularly with coexistent HIV infection. The disease is transmitted by airborne droplets when someone with the active disease coughs, talks or sneezes. Those at risk for contracting TB are persons who spend a lot of time, particularly indoors, with individuals who have active infectious tuberculosis.

The mycobacterium is covered with protective waxes and fatty substances, and is thus more durable and difficult to eradicate than many other infectious organisms. The bacteria lodge in the lungs, particularly the upper lobe, then migrate to the lymph nodes where an immune response occurs, mobilizing defenses which wall off the bacteria. Ninety-five percent of those infected with TB are successful in "locking away" the bacillus organisms, which are then incapable of growing and multiplying (Benenson, 1990). Those with 'latent' (inactive) TB are not ill and cannot infect others. However, there is an overall lifetime risk of one in ten of developing active TB later in life, particularly when immunity declines. Someone with latent TB will have a positive skin (Mantoux) test, which is a test for the presence of antibodies against the Mycobacterium organism. Many physicians recommend that someone with a reactive skin test receive preventative (prophylactic) antibiotic treatment to destroy the TB bacilli and minimize the risk of developing active TB later in life. The most common prophylactic treatment is a six to twelve month course of the medication Isoniazid.

Five percent of those infected with TB are unable to mount a successful immune response, and thus develop an active case of tuberculosis (Benenson, 1990). Those at greatest risk are infants, adolescents, and young adults. Common symptoms of the illness include fatigue, weight loss, lethargy, decreased appetite, low grade fever and night sweats. A cough generally develops slowly. Eighty-five percent of TB infections involve the lung (pulmonary tuberculosis), destroying healthy tissue in the process, however the disease can be spread through the bloodstream to many other parts of the body including the central nervous system, bones, joints, kidneys, uterus, heart, intestines and skin. In progressive pulmonary TB, approximately one half of untreated individuals will die. Overall, five to ten percent of patients die despite treatment due to drug-resistant disease, poor medication compliance, or improper drug therapy.

As mentioned previously, the rates of TB infection have risen over the past decade. Reasons for the increased incidence of this disease in the United States include HIV infection, which attacks the immune system and allows a latent infection to reactivate, the emergence of drug-resistant forms of Mycobacteria, immigration into the U.S. from countries with a high prevalence of TB infection, and social conditions which foster increased risk of transmission such as poverty, drug and alcohol abuse and homelessness.

Active TB is diagnosed with a chest x-ray, culture and microscopic examination of sputum samples. The sputum culture not only identifies the causative organism, but also allows for determination of drug sensitivity or resistance.

Treatment for the active form of tuberculosis consists of a combination of medications due to the difficulty in destroying the organisms and the presence of drug resistant forms. The combination of choice for treatment of active disease includes the medications Isoniazid, Rifampin and Pyrazinamide for approximately six months. If the organism is resistant to Isoniazid, then Ethambutol or Streptomycin is added. If HIV infection is present, a longer course of treatment is often required.

Treatment failure is usually due to irregularity in taking medications, which can foster the development of drug-resistant strains. Nationwide, fifteen percent of active TB cases are resistant to one medication and three percent are resistant to two medications. It is thus imperative that those who are treated take their full course of medication as prescribed. It is also important to be cautious when exposed to someone with active TB while they remain contagious.

Mononucleosis

Mononucleosis, also known as "The Kissing Disease" because it is transmitted by saliva exchange, is primarily a self-limited (one that does not need treatment and will go away on its own) infection of young adults. The majority of cases occur in the 15 to 30 year age range. This disease is most frequent-

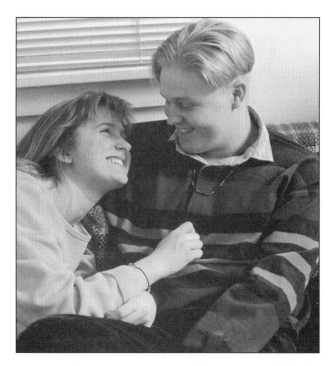

ly caused by the Epstein-Barr virus (EBV), however other viruses including cytomegalovirus (CMV) and the bacterium Toxoplasma gondii have been implicated (McCance and Huether, 1994). The offending virus attacks lymphocytes (cells found in blood and lymph tissues), which causes proliferation of cells in the immune system. This results in swelling of the lymph nodes, which is a prominent feature of this illness. After infection, there is an incubation period of thirty to fifty days (McCance and Huether, 1994). Initially, there are mild symptoms of headache and fatigue. This is followed by fever, lymph node enlargement (primarily those in the back of the neck), and sore throat, which is the most common symptom and can be quite severe.

Enlargement of the spleen (splenomegaly) can occur in up to one half of affected individuals. Rarely, this enlargement leads to the rupture of the spleen, which can be a life-threatening medical emergency. Other rare but possible complications include hepatitis, meningitis, encephalitis and coma (McCance and Huether, 1994). By far, however, the most common course is a self-limiting illness with sore throat, fatigue and fever as the principal manifestations and recovery within a few weeks.

Diagnosis is made with a blood test called the monospot agglutination test, which is specific for infection with the Epstein-Barr virus. There is also an elevation of white blood cells with a relative in-

crease in the percentage of lymphocytes and monocytes (types of white blood cells) as well as the presence of large, irregular shaped cells called atypical lymphocytes. Up to ninety-five percent of infected persons have elevated liver function tests as well.

Treatment is non-specific, including bed rest, adequate hydration and non-aspirin analgesics for pain relief. Aspirin should be avoided due to an association with Reye's Syndrome, a potentially serious complication. Sore throat pain can be decreased with salt-water gargle. Participation in contact sports should be avoided for up to one month after recovery to reduce the risk of spleen rupture. Fifteen to twenty percent of EBV antibody positive healthy adults become long-term carriers (Benenson, 1990).

Hepatitis

Hepatitis means "inflammation of the liver." There are various causes, such as alcohol or drug induced inflammation, however the most common cause of hepatitis is infection with a virus. At the current time, there are six types of viruses known to cause hepatitis (A, B, C, D, E and G) (Schering Corp., 1998). Descriptions of hepatitis have been found by Hippocrates as far back as the fifth century B.C. The first recorded cases were believed to be transmitted by the smallpox vaccine contaminated with infected human lymph tissue given to German shipyard workers in 1883 (Atkinson, et al., 1995).

The liver is the largest internal organ, with a weight of approximately three pounds. Essential to life, the liver performs multiple important functions, one of which is to clear various substances from the blood. These include medications and potential toxins, either ingested (i.e. alcohol) or manufactured in the body (such as ammonia). The liver also manufactures proteins necessary for bodily functions and stores sugar, fats and vitamins.

Viral hepatitis is a major public health concern. At the present time in the United States, over 5,000,000 people are infected with Hepatitis B or C (Schering Corp., 1999). Annually over 150,000 cases of Hepatitis C are diagnosed in this country. Nationwide 4,000,000 persons are infected with Hepatitis C, which is responsible for 8,000 to 10,000 deaths annually. This death rate is expected to triple over the next one to two decades, exceeding deaths due to AIDS. Liver failure secondary to Hepatitis C is the number one cause for liver transplantation in the United States.

The course of hepatitis can vary from asymptomatic infection (which is completely cleared by the immune system and unknown to the infected person) to rapid liver failure and death, or a slower process with cirrhosis and/or liver cancer. In early hepatitis there is an inflammation of the liver due to the response of the immune system in an attempt to eradicate the virus. The damaged liver can produce scar tissue as it attempts to heal itself, which can lead to cirrhosis (causing the liver to shrink and harden). This makes the liver unable to perform its life-sustaining functions. The individual who is chronically infected with hepatitis B or C is at a higher risk for the development of liver cancer. Unfortunately, chronic hepatitis is often asymptomatic until irreversible liver damage has occurred (Schering Corp., 1999).

As mentioned previously, there are six known types of viral hepatitis. Hepatitis A, B and C are the most common and will be covered more indepth. Whereas Hepatitis D, E and G are not as common and will only be touched upon. Hepatitis A and B are more likely to cause symptoms, whereas the B and C types are more likely to contribute to long-term health problems.

Hepatitis A

Hepatitis A poses the least serious threat to the long-term health of infected individuals. Infection is almost always acute (lasts less than six months), and the virus is generally cleared from the body by the immune system within three to four months. There is very little risk of long-term liver damage. There are no chronic carriers of Hepatitis A, as there are with B and C (Crowley, 1992).

Hepatitis A is transmitted by contact with food or water which has been contaminated with infected human waste or by direct person-to-person transmission in settings such as day care centers or institutional settings (i.e. group homes for mentally retarded individuals), where there is frequent close contact among clients and caretakers. In the US, 150,000 people are infected each year with Hepatitis A (American Liver Foundation, 1996). After exposure, the incubation period is thirty days (McCance and Huether, 1994). An infected person is contagious during the ten to fourteen days prior to symptoms and during the first week of symptoms. Antibodies develop four weeks after infection (McCance and Huether, 1994).

There may be no symptoms at all, but more commonly there is a 'flu-like' syndrome with fatigue, nausea, vomiting and upper right side abdominal pain. The course of illness varies, from mild symptoms lasting one to two weeks to severe symptoms that last for several months, although severe prolonged illness is rare (Benenson, 1990). Less often an infected person may experience fever, darkening of the urine and light-colored stools. Those at higher risk for contracting Hepatitis A are household or sexual contacts of infected individuals, children in day care settings and their adult caretaker, patients and caretakers in institutionalized settings, as well as recent travelers to developing countries.

Diagnosis is made by testing the blood and finding elevated liver enzymes and detecting antibodies against Hepatitis A. There is no specific treatment other than symptomatic, such as giving analgesics for pain and intravenous fluids in the presence of excessive vomiting to prevent dehydration. Alcohol consumption should be avoided to reduce the risk of liver damage.

A vaccine is available for this disease. The CDC recommends that persons who plan to travel to a country with poor sanitation be vaccinated approximately one month prior to travel, and repeated every four to six months if exposure continues. A vaccine is not available for general use (Benenson, 1990).

Prevention consists of proper sanitation, including careful hand washing, proper sewage disposal and effective water treatment present in developed countries. Close contacts of infected persons can help prevent infection if given immune globulin (concentrated antibodies) within two weeks of exposure (Benenson, 1990).

See Chapter five for more information on Hepatitis B

Hepatitis C

Hepatitis C is the most serious viral hepatitis to date, as mentioned earlier, affecting 4,000,000 Americans (Schering Corp., 1998). There are 30,000 new cases per year in the United States. The disease was contracted through blood transfusions given prior to 1992 (prior to the development of techniques to detect the presence of the virus in donor blood). IV drug abuse is an important risk factor for transmission of this virus; Hepatitis C transmission is very similar to that of the Hepatitis

B virus. The incubation period is 35 to 60 days (McCance and Huether, 1994) and antibodies may not appear for several months.

Most persons who contract the virus have no symptoms. Some will have the typical 'flu-like' symptoms discussed in the previous section. Eighty-five percent of those infected will develop a chronic infection, (Schering Corp., 1998) which, if untreated, places the infected person at a high risk of cirrhosis (25%), liver failure and liver cancer.

Diagnosis is made by testing liver enzyme levels and for the presence of Hepatitis C antibodies, which indicates exposure, but does not ascertain whether the infection is current. The Hepatitis C virus RNA test detects the presence of the virus in the blood.

If the infection continues beyond six months, medical treatment may be begun to decrease the risk of liver damage. Interferon (see Hepatitis B) is given for 12 to 24 months, and is effective in approximately 20–30% of cases (Microsoft Encarta, 1998). In those who do not respond to Interferon, treatment with Rebetron (a combination of Interferon and the antiviral agent Ribavirin) may be instituted. Hepatitis C virus is eliminated with this treatment in a number of patients.

There is currently no vaccine available for Hepatitis C. There is some evidence that treatment with immune globulin may prevent infection after exposure.

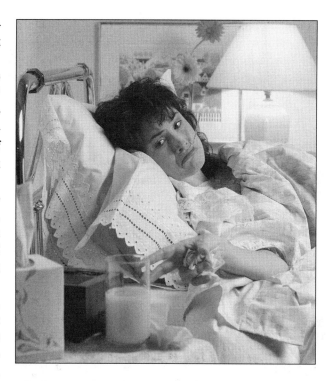

Hepatitis D, E, and G

Hepatitis D is a viral parasite, or incomplete virus, which is active only in the presence of a coexistent Hepatitis B infection. Hepatitis E is spread through contaminated food and water, much like Hepatitis A, but is not seen in the U.S. Hepatitis G has been recently identified, and there will likely be additional types characterized in future years.

Once infected, one can become contagious to others in as little as two weeks. As individuals with hepatitis are often without symptoms, it is important to be tested if exposed to the viruses. The diseases can only be correctly identified with blood tests.

A diagnosis of hepatitis is of course alarming. However, with advances in treatment, there can be optimism for recovery particularly if treatment is begun earlier in the course of the illness. Responsibility for one's health in following through with testing and receiving treatment can reduce the menace posed to public health by these illnesses. It is also important that responsible action be taken in one's conduct with others, either with self protection to prevent acquiring the disease or taking measures to protect the health of one's friends and family members with the precautions discussed previously.

Common Cold

The common cold is caused by several different viruses which are spread by droplets from sneezing or coughing, or touching surfaces where the virus is present such as hands, money or door handles. Symptoms include congestion, sneezing, sore throat, coughing and a low-grade fever. There is no treatment for the common cold; however, the symptoms can be treated to help the infected individual feel more comfortable until the virus has run its course. Gargle with salt water at the onset to relieve symptoms and possibly reduce the severity of the illness.

Influenza

Influenza (Flu) is a viral infection of the nose, throat, bronchial tubes and lungs. The flu is spread in a similar manner as the common cold. Symptoms include high fever, chills, headache, muscle and joint ache, coughing and fatigue. As with the common cold, there is no treatment for the flu; however, medication can be taken to ease the symptoms.

The following reduce the risk of contracting colds and/or flu:

Wash hands often

Keep hands away from your eyes, nose and mouth

Drink at least eight glasses of water a day

Get enough rest (6–8 hours a day)

Use kleenex instead of handkerchiefs

Get enough vitamin C

Receive a flu shot

Non-communicable Diseases

Non-communicable diseases are not transmitted person to person. These diseases can develop from many sources, some of which include genetic predisposition, behaviors such as excessive sun exposure, smoking, unhealthy eating habits and/or lack of exercise.

Cancer

Cancer is characterized by the spread of abnormal cells that serve no useful purpose. Tumors can be either benign, having a slow and expanding type of growth rate, remaining localized, and being well differentiated; or malignant, growing rapidly, infiltrating (crowding out and replacing normal cells), metastasizing (spreading to other parts of the body via the circulatory or lymphatic system) and being poorly differentiated. There are four classifications of cancers according to the type of cell and organ of origination:

Carcinoma cancers originate in epithelium (layers of cells that cover the body and line organs and glands). These are the most common.

Sarcomas begin in the supporting or connective tissues including bones, muscles and blood vessels.

Leukemias arise in the blood-forming tissues of bone marrow and spleen.

Lymphomas form in the lymphatic system.

Risk factors include a family history, race and culture, viruses, environmental and occupational hazards, cigarette smoking, alcohol consumption, poor dietary habits and psychological factors that compromise the immune system. Heredity or family history is thought to account for 10% of all cancers with the most likely sites for inherited cancers involving the breast, brain, blood, muscles, bones and adrenal glands. Research has revealed a variety of internal and external agents that are believed to cause cancer. These agents are termed carcinogens and include occupational pollutants (nickel, chromate and asbestos), chemicals in food and water, certain viruses and radiation (including the sun). The seven warning signs of cancer are:

1. Change in bowel or bladder habits
2. A sore that does not heal
3. Unusual bleeding or discharge
4. Thickening or lump in the breast, testes or elsewhere
5. Indigestion or difficulty swallowing
6. Obvious change in a wart or mole
7. Nagging cough or hoarseness

Be certain to contact a physician if you experience any of these signs (American Cancer Society).

With any cancer, early detection is the key to treatment and survival. A common misconception is that cancer is a death sentence. However, the forms of cancer with the highest incidence and mortality rates are those directly related to lifestyle factors that can be changed or eliminated. Due to dramatic improvements in diagnosis and treatment, more cancer patients are being cured and their quality of life is greatly improved. Treatment usually involves one or the combination of the following procedures:

Surgery—removal of the tumor and surrounding tissue

Radiation—X-rays which are aimed at the tumor to destroy or stop the growth.

Chemotherapy—an intravenous administration of 50 or more drugs combined to kill the cancerous cells

Immunotherapy—activating the body's own immune system with interferon injections to fight the cancerous cells

Eighty to ninety percent of all cancers are thought to be caused by environmental factors that could be prevented by either avoiding certain substances or using protective substances or devices. Healthy lifestyle practices such as not smoking

[30.5% of all cancer deaths are attributed to smoking (Harras, Edwards, Blot and Reis, 1996); those smoking two or more packs a day are 15–25 times more likely to die of cancer than nonsmokers (Hales, 1999)], exercising regularly and avoiding sun exposure are simple yet essential ways to decrease your risk of cancer. A diet low in fat (less than 30% of total calories) but high in fruits, vegetables (at least five servings per day) and whole grains is the best nutritionally for reducing cancer risk. Avoid smoke-filled areas. Second-hand or environmental tobacco smoke can increase the risk among non-smokers. Researchers have found the risk of cancer to increase threefold with as little as three hours of exposure per day (Robinson and Speer, 1995). Avoid environmental carcinogens whenever possible. Follow safety precautions if employed in or living near factories that create smoke or dust.

Skin Cancer

There are approximately 600,000 new cases of skin cancer each year. Overexposure to the ultraviolet (UV) rays of the sun is the primary culprit in these cases. Ninety percent occur on parts of the body not usually covered with clothes, including the face, hands, forearms and ears. The two most common types of skin cancers are basal cell carcinoma and squamous cell carcinoma. Both are usually treated successfully with surgery, especially if detected early. Subsequent tumors are likely in persons previously treated for these types of cancer. The fatality rate for these cancers is less than one percent.

A less prevalent but much more serious type of skin cancer is malignant melanoma and its incidence is rising 4–5% each year (Hales, 1999). This type of cancer strikes more than 40,000 and kills nearly 7,500 Americans annually (Floyd, Mimms, Yelding-Howard, 1998). Although the overall risk is 1 in 120, individuals with any of the following characteristics are at greater risk:

- Blond or red hair
- Marked freckling on upper back
- Rough red bumps on the skin (actinic keratoses)
- Family history of melanoma
- Three or more blistering sunburns during the teenage years

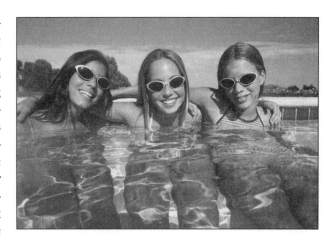

- Three or more years at an outdoor summer job during the teenage years
- Living in the southern United States

A person's risk increases three to four times with one or two of the factors listed above. With three or more, the risk is increased to 20 to 25 times (Marwick, 1995).

Occupational exposure to carcinogens and inherited skin disorders are risk factors as well. Malignant melanomas are highly curable if detected early, however the chance of recurrence is high. To help prevent skin cancer: avoid the sun anytime your shadow is shorter than you are, cover up when in the sun (wear wide-brimmed hats, long sleeves and pants), use a sunscreen with a Sun Protection Factor (SPF) of at least 15; beware of cloudy days (when burning is still possible), water (the sun's rays can reach 3 feet deep) and snow (which reflects sunlight). Avoid use of tanning beds or sunlamps. "Tanning beds are potentially even more dangerous than the actual sun because of the concentrated effect of the bulbs. The concentrated UV radiation from the bulbs makes a few minutes in a tanning bed equal to several hours in the sun" (Spence, 1998). Observe your skin for changes in size, color, number and thickness of moles, or pigmented growths, spots or changes in birthmarks.

Monthly Skin Self-Exam (SSE) can reveal cancerous changes at an early stage. Use a systematic approach. During this exam, one looks for abnormal growth of cells. To begin, start with the head and work downward. Use a hair dryer on a cool setting to move hair out of the way to allow examination of the scalp more easily. Abnormal growth would be characterized by changes in:

- size—a sudden or continuous enlargement.
- shape—the development of irregular margins.
- color—multiple shades of dark brown or black.
- elevation—when a previously flat mole rises higher than the surrounding skin.
- texture—when the mole becomes soft or looks crumbly.
- sensation—when the mole becomes itchy, tender or painful.

If you notice any of these warning signs see your physician immediately.

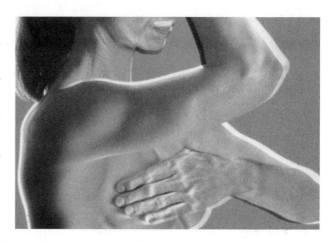

Lung Cancer

Lung cancer is the number one cause of cancer deaths in the U.S. (Harras et al., 1996). The major cause of lung cancer is cigarette smoking, accounting for 85% of all lung cancer deaths, making it one of the most preventable forms of cancer. Smoking cessation would decrease the death rate of lung cancer in half. Other risk factors include asbestos exposure, secondhand smoke, radiation exposure and radon exposure. Early detection of lung cancer is difficult, resulting in only 15% of cases being discovered early. With early detection, there is a 43% chance of surviving twelve months; however, the overall five-year relative survival rate is only 13%. Symptoms include a nagging or persistent cough, blood in the sputum, chest pain, shortness of breath, recurring bronchitis or pneumonia, weight loss, loss of appetite and/or anemia.

Breast Cancer

Among women in the U.S., breast cancer is the most common form of cancer (other than skin) and is a leading cause of cancer mortality (Harras et al., 1996). Risk factors include: age 40 years or older, family history or personal history of breast cancer, early onset of menstruation, having no children, having a first child at a late age (after 30), late menopause, exposure to radiation, obesity (for postmenopausal women) and certain types of benign breast disease (premenopausal women). Early detection is the best way to reduce the mortality rate among breast cancer patients. It is recommended by the American Cancer Society that women 20 years of age and older perform a breast self-examination once a month. Any persistent lumps, swelling, thickening or distortion of the breast, pain or tenderness of the nipple, or discharge of blood or fluid from the nipple should be reported immediately. A diagnostic X-ray, called a mammogram, can detect a tumor two or three years before it can be detected by a self-exam. The ACS recommends all women begin routine mammograms by the age of 40, and physicians recommend that women at high risk (with a family history) have mammograms every 6 to 12 months beginning between the ages of 25 and 35. With early diagnosis and a localized tumor, there is a 97% chance of surviving 5 years.

Breast Self-Exam (BSE) is a method utilized in an effort to promptly detect lumps located in the breast. During this exam, one looks for masses within the soft tissue of the breast or changes in the breast appearance. Due to the varying texture, size, and sensitivity of one's breast, it is important to do the self-exam at the same time each month. The following is a guideline to determine the proper timing:

Women with menstrual cycles—one week after the beginning of the menstrual period when the breasts are usually not tender.

After menopause or hysterectomy—choose a day that is easy to remember, such as the first day of the month.

Procedures:

Step One: Mirror

Stand in front of a mirror and examine your breasts from the front and side. Look for any changes in the form, shape, signs of dimpling or puckering, scaling or discharge from the nipple.

TABLE 6.1 Recommended Breast Exam Schedule

Procedure	Risk	Age	Frequency
Breast Self-Exam	Average	20 & Over	Once a Month
	High*	20 & Over	Once a Month
Breast Exam by Clinician	Average	20 to 39	Every 3 Years
	Average	40 & Over	Every Year
	High*	20 to 39	Every Year
Mammography	Average	40 & Over	Once a Year
	High*	Begin between 25 & 35	Once Every 6–12 Months

*Personal history of breast cancer or family history of premenopausal breast cancer in mother or sister.

Step Two: Bath or Shower

As you are examining your breasts you are feeling for a lump, a thickened area, a hardening in the breast or anything that feels different. Place one hand behind your head. With your other hand, press flat fingers gently in small circular motions. Begin with your index finger next to your collarbone. Move your hand in a circular fashion clockwise around the breast. You will feel a ridge of tissue in the lower curve of your breast; this is normal. When you reach the top of your breast, move in three fingers and continue examining your breast with the same circular motion. Continue this process until you reach the nipple. Repeat this procedure with your other breast.

Step Three: Lying Down

Examining your breasts while lying on your back is the most effective way to check your breast for lumps, thickening or hardening.

Lie flat on your back with your left arm over your head and a pillow or folded towel under your left shoulder. With your right hand, press flat fingers gently in small circular motions. Begin with your index finger next to your collarbone. Move your hand in a circular fashion clockwise around the breast. You will feel the ridge of tissue in the lower curve of your breast. When you reach the top of your breast, move in three fingers and continue as before, until you reach the nipple. Repeat these steps with your other breast. You can use lotion or powder on the skin, which will allow your fingers to slide smoothly.

If you notice a change in your breasts, see your doctor or health care provider promptly. Important changes to report include:

- a lump, thickening or hardening in your breast
- dimpling or puckering of the skin on your breast
- scaling of the skin around the nipple
- nipple discharge

(American Cancer Society)

Cervical Cancer

Cervical cancer is representative of abnormal growth and maturation of the cervical squamous epithelium. Typically there are no symptoms in the early stages. Eventually individuals with cervical cancer will have uterine bleeding, cramps, infections and pain in the abdominal region. Risk factors include: first vaginal intercourse at an early age, multiple sexual partners, cigarette smoking and infections with certain types of human papilloma viruses. The Pap Smear is a screening test a physician performs in order to check for pre-cancerous cells or early cancer of the cervix. The physician obtains a sampling of tissue from inside the cervix and sends the specimen to a lab to be analyzed. Due to early detection with the Pap smear, cancer of the cervix is rare and is easily treated in women

CHART 6.1 Cancer Related Checkups

Following are guidelines for the early detection of cancer in people without symptoms. Talk with your doctor—ask how these guidelines relate to you. Remember these guidelines are not rules and apply only to people without symptoms. If you have any of the seven warning signals of cancer, see your doctor or go to your clinic without delay.

Age 20 to 40: Cancer-Related Checkup Every 3 Years

Should include the procedures listed below plus health counseling (such as tips on quitting smoking) and examinations for cancers of the thyroid, testes, prostate, mouth, ovaries, skin and lymph nodes. Some people are at higher risk for certain cancers and may need to have tests more frequently.

Breast
- Examination by doctor every three years
- Self-exam every month
- One baseline mammogram between ages 35 and 40

Higher risk for breast cancer: personal or family history of breast cancer, never had children and/or first child after 30

Uterus
- Pelvic exam every three years

Cervix
- Pap smear after three initial negative tests one year apart—at least every three years (includes women under 18 if sexually active)

Higher risk for cervical cancer: early age at first intercourse and/or multiple sex partners

Testes
- Self-exam every month
- Consult doctor when an abnormality is present

Higher risk for testicular cancer: personal or family history of testicular cancer, undescended testicles not corrected during early childhood and/or Caucasian under age 35

Age 40 and Over: Cancer-Related Checkup Every Year

Should include the procedures listed here, plus health counseling, (such as tips on quitting smoking) and examinations for cancers of the thyroid, testes, prostate, mouth, ovaries, skin and lymph nodes. Some people are at higher risk for certain cancers and may need to have tests more frequently

Breast
- Examinations by doctor every year
- Self-exam every month
- Mammogram every year after age 40

Higher risk for breast cancer: personal or family history of breast cancer, never had children and/or first child after 30

Uterus
- Pelvic examination every year

Cervix
- Pap smear after two initial negative tests one year apart—at least every three years

Higher risk for cervical cancer: early age at first intercourse and/or multiple sex partners

Endometrium
- Endometrial tissue sample at menopause if at risk

Higher risk for endometrial cancer: infertility, obesity, failure of ovulation, abnormal uterine bleeding and/or estrogen therapy

Colon and Rectum
- Digital rectal examination every year
- Guaiac slide test every year after age 50
- Procto exam—after two initial negative tests one year apart—every three to five years after age 50

Higher risk for colorectal cancer: personal or family history of colon or rectal cancer, personal or family history of polyps in the colon or rectum, ulcerative colitis

Prostate
- Digital rectal examination and PSA test every year

Higher risk for prostate cancer: a history of previous urinary tract infections and over age 50

---

who have regular exams. It is recommended that all females over 18 or who have had sexual intercourse have a Pap smear annually. This procedure should continue until an individual reaches the age of 70, at which point the physician may recommend discontinuing Pap smears. The best time to schedule a pap smear is 14 days after the start of a period. Do not have intercourse for 24 hours or any substances in the vagina for 48 hours before the exam.

Testicular Cancer

Although testicular cancer accounts for only 3% of cancers of the male genitals and urinary tract, it is one of the most common cancers in young males, with the majority of cases identified between the ages of 15 and 34 (American Cancer Society). Men with undescended testicles in childhood seem to be at greatest risk. Other risks may include: family history, inguinal hernia, testicular trauma, mumps orchitis, elevated testicular temperature, vasectomy or exposure to electromagnetic fields. Testicular self-exams should be performed monthly to detect any enlargement or thickening of the testes. The cure rate if detected early is close to 80%.

Testicular Self-Exam (TSE) can detect cancer in early stages when disease is more curable. Exams should begin at age 15. Self-examination should be performed every month in order to detect any changes. The best time to perform the exam is after taking a warm bath or shower when the skin of the scrotum is relaxed.

Procedures:

Step One: Mirror
Examine the scrotum visually for swelling or a change in consistency.

Step Two: After a Bath or Shower
Roll each testicle gently between the thumb and fingers of both hands. If you find any lumps, nodules or swelling within a testicle you should see your doctor promptly.

(American Cancer Society)

Colon and Rectum Cancer

Colon and Rectum cancer are the third leading type of cancer in men and women, claiming about 60,000 lives a year (Hales, 1999). The majority of cases occur in men and women over the age of 50. Risk factors include a family or personal history of colorectal cancer or polyps (growths) and ulcerative colitis. High fat, low-fiber diets have also been shown to increase the risk. Symptoms include bleeding from the rectum, blood in the stool, or a change in bowel habits (recurring constipation or diarrhea). Digital rectal exams, stool blood tests and proctoscopic exams can detect early stages of colorectal cancer. It is recommended that a digital rectal exam is performed annually after age 40, a stool blood test performed every year after age 50 and a proctosigmoidoscopy performed every 3 to 5 years after age 50. Regular exercise has been shown to re-duce the risk in both men and women (Lee, et al., 1991). Hormone replacement therapy in post-menopausal women may significantly lower the risk of colon cancer.

Oral Cancers

Oral cancers (cancers of the lip, tongue, mouth and pharynx) account for almost 4% of all malignancies in the U.S. (Boring, Squires, Tong et al., 1994). In 1994 30,000 new cases were reported and approximately 7,900 people died of the disease. Oral cancer is related directly to a person's behavior. The major behavioral risk factors include cigarette, pipe or cigar smoking, excessive alcohol use, and tobacco use. Particularly vulnerable are persons who drink and smoke. Early symptoms include: a bleeding sore that will not heal, a lump or thickening, a red or white patch (lesion) that will not go away, a persistent sore throat, difficulty chewing, swallowing or moving of the tongue or jaws. A cure is often achieved easily with early detection.

Asthma

Asthma is a respiratory disorder which involves difficulty breathing, wheezing and/or coughing due to the constriction of the bronchial tubes. An individual will typically notice a wheezing sound when they are trying to breathe, while coughing and/or when experiencing difficulty breathing. In some cases those who suffer from asthma can stop an attack by simply removing themselves from an irritant such as cigarette smoke. Most of the time asthma attacks require some type of medical intervention and in rare cases, death can result from lack of treatment. Antihistamines, corticosteroids, and bronchodilating drugs are usually successful in reducing the bronchospasm. Reducing exposure to allergens, such as air pollution, pollen, dust, secondhand smoke, animal fur, bee venom, and specific foods, as well as nonallergens such as stress or intense exercise can help prevent further asthma attacks. In the event that one must encounter an irritant, prescription drugs are available that help prevent asthma attacks. Some individuals are more likely to have difficulties with asthma: those with a family history, presence of atopy (the predisposition to respond to environmental allergens with specific IgE antibody production), exposure to allergens, certain viral infections and cigarette smoke (Morley, 1991). Children whose mothers smoke at least half a pack of cigarettes a day are

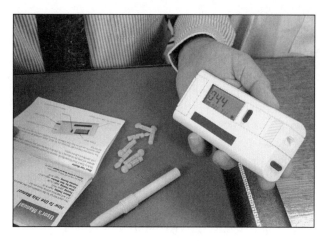

twice as likely to have asthma as children of non-smoking mothers (University of California, Berkley). Approximately one out of twenty people have asthma (Monismith and Olsen, 1996). More children than adults suffer from asthma, because many children outgrow this condition.

Diabetes

Diabetes is the result of insufficient insulin production or the body's inability to utilize insulin readily produced by the pancreas. Insulin has two major functions: to move glucose from the blood to the cells of the body where it is used as energy and to convert excess glucose to glycogen, for storage as an energy reserve in the liver and the muscles for later use (Floyd, et al., 1998). There are two types of diabetes, Type I and Type II.

Type I or insulin dependent diabetes is typically associated with child or adolescent onset. In this form of diabetes the pancreas does not produce insulin, and the individual requires regular injections. The signs and symptoms of Type I diabetes appear suddenly and dramatically. Symptoms include fatigue, irritability, abnormal hunger and thirst, frequent urination, and weight loss (Floyd, et al., 1998). This type of diabetes is only seen in about 5% of all diabetics and is considered the more serious of the two forms.

Type II or non-insulin dependent diabetes is typically associated with adult onset and obesity. In this form of the disease the pancreas produces insulin, but the cells of the body are not able to use it effectively. The onset of Type II diabetes is more gradual than Type I. Some symptoms include drowsiness, blurred vision, itching, slow healing of cuts, skin infections, and numbness of fingers or toes (Floyd, et al., 1998).

If an individual suffering from diabetes is not treated, the illness can progress into a diabetic coma. If too much insulin is taken or inadequate food is eaten, an insulin reaction may occur, which if serious, can result in a seizure (convulsion). Patients with diabetes have a higher incidence of arteriosclerosis and the associated complications such as strokes, heart attacks, and gangrene of the lower extremities due to poor circulation, as well as degenerative effects of the small blood vessels supplying the retina of the eye which can lead to blindness.

The goal for those who have this condition is to balance blood sugar levels. This can be done with insulin regimens, a structured diet and regular exercise. With type I diabetes, the individual usually can achieve this by monitoring the blood glucose level and adjusting the amount of insulin injected each day. In type II diabetes, this can be accomplished with a controlled diet and regular exercise alone; in some instances oral hypoglycemic medication or insulin is required as well. The risk of developing diabetes can be reduced with regular activity, which reduces body weight and fat levels, and increases insulin sensitivity and glucose tolerance (Sharkey, 1997). Healthy dietary habits also decrease the fat levels as well as obesity, therefore enhancing the body's ability to transport glucose into the muscles.

Approximately one out of twenty Americans have diabetes (American Diabetes Association). Diabetes is the leading cause of blindness among adults and accounts for about half of all amputations annually (Monismith, et al., 1996).

Anemia

Anemia means "without blood". It is a condition in which the quantity or quality of red blood cells is insufficient. Normal red blood cells contain hemoglobin which carries oxygen to organs and tissues. Anemic individuals have a reduced oxygen-carrying capacity. Anemias can be the result of too little iron, loss of blood (including heavy menstrual bleeding or frequent blood donations), insufficient red-cell production or genetic abnormalities. Symptoms include fatigue, infection and/or trouble healing. There are four types of anemias known:

Iron-deficiency anemia—develops with inadequate iron intake in the diet or excessive loss of iron, which can result from heavy menses. This is the most common form of anemia and can be corrected with iron supplements.

Pernicious anemia—caused by deficiency of vitamin B12, which decreases the production of red blood cells. The deficiency is due to an inability of the body to absorb B12 and is treated with vitamin B12 injections.

Aplastic anemia—stems from bone marrow failure resulting in a decreased number of red blood cells. Injury to bone marrow usually results from ingesting a toxic drug or chemical. Treatment is primarily with blood transfusions; however, the condition is most often fatal.

Sickle-cell anemia—an inherited trait caused by abnormal hemoglobins. These abnormal hemoglobins cause the red blood cells to be sickle-shaped, which impedes the flow of oxygen-carrying blood. Signs and symptoms include episodes of severe pain, swelling in hands or feet, susceptibility to infection due to a weakened immune system and possible premature death. There is no cure for sickle-cell anemia, although the cancer drug hydroxyurea has proved to be successful in alleviating the pain. Sickle-cell anemia affects approximately 72,000 African Americans and one out of every 1,000–1,500 Hispanics in the U.S. (Floyd et al., 1998). This type of anemia is a recessive trait-inherited condition, so there are many asymptomatic carriers without the disease. Because of this and the fact that there is no cure, the emphasis is shifting to prevention through education and genetic counseling.

Gastrointestinal Disorders

Ulcers, which are open sores, can develop in the lining of the stomach (gastric ulcers) or small intestine (duodenal ulcers) and are due to the corrosive effect of excessive gastric juices. Conventional theory blames lifestyle factors such as stress and diet. However, new research has identified a link between the bacterium Helicobacter pylori (H. pylori) and the formation of ulcers. One theory suggests that an infection caused by this bacteria leads to an inflammation of the stomach lining which results in increased susceptibility of the stomach to stressors such as smoking, alcohol, high fat diets and/or anxiety. The most prominent symptom is a burning pain in the upper abdomen that is related to the digestive cycle. A bleeding ulcer, although not common, can be fatal. Excessive weight loss and anemia can result from an untreated ulcer. Medications that reduce stomach acid and relieve symptoms, lifestyle changes such as eating small, frequent meals, avoiding high-fat foods, cigarettes, alcohol, caffeine and taking antacids can all reduce the effects of ulcers. One in five men and one in ten women suffer from peptic ulcers. Risk factors include: a stressful lifestyle, cigarette smoking, heavy use of alcohol, caffeine or painkillers containing aspirin or ibuprofen, advanced age and family history.

Irritable Bowel Syndrome (spastic colon or irritable colon) is a very common problem resulting from intestinal spasms. Symptoms include episodes of abdominal cramping, nausea, pain, gas, loud gurgling bowel sounds, and disturbed bowel function. No biochemical or structural abnormalities have been identified as the cause, therefore, no standard medical treatment exists for IBS. Common interventions include reducing emotional stress, eating high-fiber diets, or taking stool softeners, laxatives, and drugs to reduce intestinal spasms.

References

American Cancer Society.

American Liver Foundation. 1996. What You Should Know about Hepatitis A, B, and C. Cedar Grove, NJ.

Atkinson, W., et al. 1995. Epidemiology & Prevention of Vaccine-Preventable Diseases. 2d ed. Department of Health and Human Services. Centers for Disease Control and Prevention.

Benenson, A. *Control of Communicable Diseases in Man.* 15th ed. Washington, DC: American Public Health Association 1990.

Boring, C., et al. 1994. Cancer Statistics. CA Cancer Journal Clin. 44: 7–26.

Crowley, L. 1992. *Introduction to Human Disease.* 3d ed. Boston, MA: Jones and Bartlett Publishers, Inc.

Floyd, P., et al. *Personal Health: Perspectives and Lifestyles.* 2d ed. Englewood, CO: Morton Publishing Co 1998.

Hales, D. *An Invitation to Health,* 8th ed. Pacific Grove, CA: Brooks/Cole Publishing Co 1999.

Harras, A., et al. 1996. "Cancer Rates and Risks" National Cancer Institute (U.S.); NIH Publication no. 96-691 4th ed. http://rex.nci.nih.gov/NCI%5Fpub%5Finterface/raterisk/index.html

Lee, M., et al. 1991. Physical Activity and Risk of Developing Colorectal Cancer among College Alumni. *Journal of the National Cancer Institute*, 83: 1324–9.

Marwick, C. 1995. New Light on Skin Cancer Mechanisms. *Journal of the American Medical Association*, 274:6.

McCance, K. and Huether, S. *Pathophysiology: The Biologic Basis for Disease in Adults and Children.* 2d ed. St. Louis, Missouri: Mosby-Year Book, Inc 1994.

Microsoft Encarta. 1998.

Monismith, S. and Olsen, L. *An Introduction to Health and Disease*. 3d ed. Dubuque, IA: Kendall/Hunt Publishing Co 1996.

Morley, J. *Preventive Therapy in Asthma*. San Diego, CA: Academic Press Limited 1991.

Robinson, J. and Speer, T. 1995. "The Air We Breathe." *American Demographics*. 17:6.

Schering Corporation 1998. *What Everyone Should Know about Hepatitis.* Kenilworth, NJ.

Schering Corporation 1999. *Detection and Referral: The Primary Care Physician Guide to Chronic Viral Hepatitis*. Kenilworth, N.J.

Sharkey, B. *Fitness and Health*. 4th ed. Champaign, IL: Human Kinetics 1997.

Spence, W. 1998. Skin Cancer: The Bare Facts. Health Edco.

University of California, Berkley. November, 1990. Wellness Letter.

Contacts

American Cancer Society
800-ACS-2345
http://www.cancer.org

American Diabetes Association
800-342-2383
http://www.diabetes.org

American Institute for Cancer Research
http://www.aicr.org

American Liver Foundation
1425 Pompton Avenue
Cedar Grove, NJ 07009
800-223-0179

Asthma and Allergy Foundation of America
800-7-ASTHMA
http://www.AAFA.org

Asthma Information Line
800-822-2762
http://www.nhlbi.nih.gov/nhlbi/nhlbi/.htm

Cancer Information Service
800-4-CANCER
http://cancernet.nci.nih.gov/

Center for Disease Control and Prevention
http://www.cdc.gov

InfoTex 979-268-0378
(Enter any 4-digit code below when prompted.)
7104 Cancer warning signs
7108 Cancer risk factors
7125 Ulcers
7137 Asthma
4536 Diabetes warning signs

Juvenile Diabetes Foundation International
800-223-1138
http://www.jdfcure.com

National Headache Foundation
800-843-2256
http://www.headaches.org

National Institute of Diabetes, Digestive and Kidney Diseases
http://www.niddk.nih.gov

Notebook Activities

Develop Family Tree (up to great grandparents) What disease(s) do/did they have?

Check Your Asthma "I.Q."

Could You Have Diabetes & not Know It?

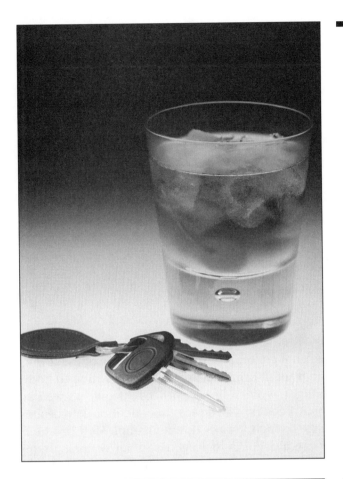

Chapter Seven

Drugs

"First we form habits, then they form us. Conquer your bad habits, or they'll eventually conquer you."

—Dr. Rob Gilbert

OBJECTIVES

Students will be able to:

- Identify types of alcoholic beverages and the alcohol content for each
- Identify the physiological and societal effects of alcohol
- Identify penalties for alcohol related offenses
- Identify factors relating to binge drinking and alcohol poisoning
- Identify risk of drinking and driving
- Identify the adverse effects of tobacco use
- Identify types of tobacco use
- Identify the effects of environmental tobacco smoke
- Identify types of psychoactive drugs and their physiological effects
- Identify the types and risks of inhalant use
- Identify the adverse effects of Rohypnol and GHB

The purpose of this chapter is to provide an overview of substance use and abuse and the detrimental effects of alcohol, tobacco and psychoactive drugs, and their effects on a healthy lifestyle.

Alcohol

Prevalence

According to the National Institute on Alcohol Abuse and Alcoholism (NIAAA), more than 60 percent of adults are regular drinkers. Currently, there are 18 million Americans experiencing problems with alcohol and 10 million are alcoholics. But, in addition to addiction and health issues, alcohol contributes to many other serious problems in our society. Some of these problems can be fatal. For example, according to the NIAAA, alcohol is a factor in:

- Over 40% of all highway deaths
- 50% of all spousal abuse cases
- 30% of child abuse cases
- 65% of drowning
- 54% of those jailed for violent crimes were intoxicated

• 49% convicted of murder or attempted murder

What Is Alcohol?

Ethyl alcohol, or ethanol, has been prevalent in our society for centuries. Except for the Prohibition in the United States from 1917 to 1932 when alcohol was considered an illegal substance, it has become the legal and accepted drug of choice. There are three major types of alcoholic beverages; beer, distilled spirits or hard liquor, and wine or wine coolers.

Distilled spirits include scotch, gin, rum, vodka, tequila, whiskey, etc. The alcohol content varies according to the proof of the beverage, which is twice the percent of alcohol. For example, if whiskey is 80 proof then that particular beverage is 40% alcohol by volume. The average mixed drink contains a 1-ounce shot of hard liquor.

Wine usually averages 12% alcohol by volume and wine coolers average approximately 5% alcohol by volume. The average glass of wine is 4 ounces, and wine coolers are usually served in 12 ounce bottles.

Beer is usually served in 12-ounce cans or bottles. The average alcohol content of beer is 4.5% by volume. To be considered a beer, the alcohol content must not exceed 5% by weight by volume. If the amount of alcohol is greater it is considered an ale.

Blood alcohol concentration (BAC) is the measure of concentration of alcohol in blood, expressed in grams per 100 ml. An example would be 100mg. of alcohol in 10ml. of blood would be reported as .10 percent.

12 oz. Beer × .045	12 oz. Wine cooler × .05
.54 oz. Alcohol	.60 oz. Alcohol
1 oz. Whiskey × .40	4 oz. Wine × .12
.40 oz. Alcohol	.48 oz. Alcohol

The alcoholic content of some other typical drinks:

1 oz. shot 86 proof liquor	.43 oz.
Light beer 12 oz.	.46 oz.
Champagne 4 oz.	.58 oz.
Malt liquor 12 oz.	.75 oz
Margarita	.75 oz

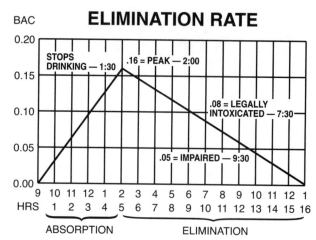

Texas Commission on Alcohol and Drug Abuse.

FIGURE 7.1

Factors influencing a person's BAC are gender, alcohol content of the drink, and size of the drink, time spent drinking, and food. In addition to body weight, women do not process alcohol as well as men because of the enzyme alcohol dehydrogenase, which breaks down alcohol. Men produce more alcohol dehydrogenase than women; therefore, men can eliminate alcohol at a slightly faster rate (Texas Commission on Alcohol and Drug Abuse, 1995). Women also have less water content, so a woman at the same weight as a man will have a higher BAC. The higher alcohol content of a drink, the higher BAC it will produce. For example, a 1 ounce shot of a 100 proof beverage has more alcohol than a 1-ounce shot of an 80 proof beverage. The larger an alcoholic drink, the more alcohol it will contain and produce a higher BAC. For example, a 24-ounce beer will have twice the amount of alcohol than a 12-ounce beer. The liver begins to process alcohol shortly after it is absorbed into the bloodstream. The longer time factor will result in a lower BAC. For example, if a person drinks a six-pack in three hours, they will have a lower BAC than if they had consumed a six-pack in one hour. Having food in the stomach may coat the lining of the stomach, therefore slowing down the absorption of alcohol. Food will not absorb or soak up the alcohol, so the alcohol will eventually reach the bloodstream.

There are three ways that alcohol is removed or eliminated from the body. Ninety percent of alcohol is eliminated through the oxidation process of the liver at .015 percent per hour. The alcohol dehydrogenase then converts alcohol to acetaldehyde. Alcohol is then metabolized at approximately .25 to .30 ounces per hour, regardless of the blood alcohol concentration. The rate of metabolism is based on the activity of alcohol dehydrogenase, working at its own pace (Ray, 1996). Eight percent of alcohol is eliminated through breath, which is why a breath test is used to determine BAC. A small amount of alcohol, approximately two percent, is eliminated through sweat. Contrary to popular belief, cold showers, black coffee, aspirin or exercise will not speed up this elimination process.

Tolerance is when an individual adapts to the amount consumed so that larger quantities are needed to achieve the same effect. This basically means that a person needs to drink more alcohol to achieve the same effect. This can take place over several months or years of consuming alcohol; depending on the amount consumed and at what age the individual begins to drink. At some point, after a person's tolerance has increased over a period of time, it begins to drop, allowing the affects of alcohol to be felt after only a few drinks. This reverse tolerance is caused by the natural aging process or liver disease after years of abusive drinking (Texas Commission on Alcohol and Drug Abuse, 1995).

Intoxication is defined as a transient state of physical and mental disruption due to the presence of a toxic substance, such as alcohol (Maisto, 1995). As BAC increases, the central nervous system alters behavior and physical function. Change can occur as low as .02 BAC in some people, while everyone is impaired to some degree at .05 BAC.

Calculating the percentage of alcohol in your bloodstream.

This table presents the approximate blood alcohol concentration (BAC) according to your body weight and the number of drinks consumed during 1 or 2 hours.

Number of Drinks	Body weight, pounds							
	100	120	140	160	180	200	220	240
For 1 hour of drinking:								
1	0.03	0.03	0.02	0.02	0.02	0.01	0.01	—
2	0.06	0.05	0.04	0.04	0.03	0.03	0.03	0.02
3	0.10	0.08	0.07	0.06	0.05	0.05	0.04	0.04
4	0.13	0.10	0.09	0.08	0.07	0.06	0.06	0.05
5	0.16	0.13	0.11	0.10	0.09	0.08	0.07	0.07
6	0.19	0.16	0.13	0.12	0.11	0.10	0.09	0.08
7	0.23	0.19	0.16	0.14	0.13	0.11	0.10	0.09
8	0.26	0.22	0.18	0.16	0.14	0.13	0.12	0.11
For 2 hours of drinking:								
1	0.01	0.01	—	—	—	—	—	—
2	0.04	0.03	0.02	0.01	0.01	0.01	—	—
3	0.08	0.06	0.04	0.03	0.03	0.02	0.02	0.01
4	0.11	0.09	0.07	0.06	0.05	0.04	0.03	0.03
5	0.15	0.12	0.10	0.08	0.07	0.06	0.05	0.04
6	0.18	0.14	0.12	0.10	0.09	0.08	0.07	0.06
7	0.22	0.18	0.15	0.12	0.11	0.09	0.08	0.07
8	0.25	0.20	0.17	0.15	0.13	0.11	0.10	0.09

Effects of blood alcohol concentrations

- *.02% BAC:* You feel a bit relaxed and loosened up. Your mood is heightened, but there is little behavior change.

- *.04% BAC:* You feel more relaxed. Your muscular coordination is slightly decreased.

- *.06% BAC:* Your judgment begins to be impaired. You may become louder and boisterous. Your speech begins to slur. You have difficulty making decisions about ability to drive or operate machinery.

- *.08% BAC: You are considered legally drunk in many places.* This is the equivalent of the BAC found in a 160-pound male drinking 4 drinks in an hour. Your balance, vision, and hearing are slightly impaired. You are talkative and noisy. Your muscular coordination and driving skills are affected. Four hours will be required for alcohol to disappear from your system.

- *.10% BAC: You are legally drunk in most places.* Your mental facilities and judgment are distinctly impaired. Five hours will be required for all alcohol to disappear from your system.

- *.12% BAC:* This is equivalent to the BAC a 160-pound male would have if he drank a six-pack of beer in an hour. You will be distinctly clumsy and show serious lack of judgment. Vomiting may occur.

- *.14% BAC:* You're staggering, your speech is highly slurred, your vision quite blurred.

- *.16% BAC:* This is equal to a half pint of whiskey, or 8 drinks, for a 160-pound male consumed in an hour. You might as well go to bed, since it will take 8 hours for the alcohol to be metabolized through your system.

- *.20% BAC:* You'll be highly confused and will need assistance moving about. If you stop now, you'll still be legally drunk 6 hours from now.

- *.30% BAC:* This is equal to the BAC produced by a pint of whiskey consumed by a 160-pound male in an hour. Judgment and coordination are gone; the senses don't register anything and you may lose consciousness.

- *.40% BAC:* This is equal to 1¼ pints, or 20 shots, of whiskey for a 160-pound male consumed in an hour. You will lose consciousness and be in a coma. You will also be dangerously close to death—perhaps even dead. At a blood alcohol level of *.40%–.50%*, a person is usually in a coma. At *.60%–.70%*, death occurs.

From *Healthy for Life: Wellness and the Art of Living* (also: Health Information Update 1994–95), 1st Edition, by B. Williams and S. Knight. © 1994. Reprinted with permission of Wadsworth Publishing, a division of Thomson Learning. Fax 800-730-2215.

Physiological Effects of Alcohol

Alcohol is a drug that has two major effects on the body. Being a depressant it slows down the nervous system (respiratory and cardiovascular systems). Alcohol and its by-products also irritate the nerve endings and eventually sedate or deaden them. Vision is another sense that alcohol affects quickly. This is an important ability for driving because ninety percent of the information we receive is obtained through vision. Alcohol has a direct effect on our vision by causing the loss of fine muscle control in the eyes accounting for eye focus, visual acuity, peripheral vision, color distinction, night vision, distance judgment, and double vision (Texas Commission on Alcohol and Drug Abuse, 1995). Other physiological effects are impaired mental and physical reflexes, increased risk of diseases such as cancer of the brain, tongue, mouth, esophagus, larynx, liver and the bladder. Heart and blood pressure problems are also associated with alcohol consumption

Laws Relating to Alcohol

Minor in Possession (MIP)

In Texas, it is illegal for a person under the age of 21 to attempt to purchase, possess, or consume alcohol. It is also illegal to misrepresent that you are 21 or older to obtain alcohol. This offense is considered a Class C Misdemeanor and punishment can include fines up to $500, community service, loss of driver's license, alcohol awareness class, and possibly jail.

Driving Under the Influence by a minor

In Texas, it is illegal for a minor to operate a motor vehicle in a public place with *any* detectible amount of alcohol in his/her system. This may be determined by a blood/breath test or simply smelling alcohol on the minor's breath. The penalties are very similar to MIP with fine, loss of license, education courses, and community service.

Administrative License Revocation (ALR)

This law is for suspension of a minor's driver's license for failing a blood/breath test or for having a detectible amount of alcohol in his/her system.

Implied Consent

In Texas, by operating a motor vehicle in a public place, the driver has given consent to take a breath/blood test to determine alcohol in his/her system. Refusing to take the test is considered a violation and penalties can result in loss of license, regardless of the outcome of the violation.

Driving While Intoxicated

In Texas, the state defines intoxication as not having normal use of your mental or physical faculties because of alcohol or other drugs; and an alcohol concentration of .08 or more. This is a Class B Misdemeanor and first offense penalties can include fine, loss of license, jail time.

Public Intoxication

The three provisions for a Public Intoxication offense include being in a public place, intoxication, and possibly being a danger to yourself and/or others. Penalties vary.

Intoxication Assault

When someone is injured in an alcohol related accident, the intoxicated driver can be charged with Intoxication Assault, which is a third degree felony in Texas. Penalties vary.

Intoxication Manslaughter

When someone is killed as a result of drinking and driving. The intoxicated driver may be charged with intoxication manslaughter, which is a second-degree felony in Texas.

Societal Problems

The dangers of alcohol consumption are a major problem in our society. Drinking too much alcohol can cause a range of very serious problems, in addition to the obvious health issues. Alcohol is a contributing factor in motor vehicle accidents,

violence, school/work problems as well as family problems.

Motor Vehicle Accidents

Drinking and driving is one of our country's more serious problems and one that is one-hundred percent avoidable. More than 40 percent of all fatal crashes in the United States are alcohol related (NHTSA, 1998). Alcohol related crashes in the U.S. cost the public more than $110 billion in 1996. The average alcohol related fatality cost $3 million, $1.2 in monetary cost and $1.8 million in quality of life loss (NHTSA, 1998).

The NHTSA states that 15,935 people were killed in alcohol-related traffic accidents, an average of one death every 33 minutes. An estimated three in every ten Americans will be involved in an alcohol-related crash at some time in their lives. It is also estimated that every weekday night from 10:00 p.m. to 1:00 a.m., one in 13 drivers are drunk. Between 1:00 a.m. and 6:00 a.m. on weekend mornings, one in seven drivers are drunk (Miller et al., 1996). Although more Americans have died in alcohol-related crashes than all the wars the U.S. has been involved in, there has been a steady decrease in alcohol related deaths since 1982. The NHTSA estimates that between 90,307 and 128,520 lives have been saved between the years of 1983 and 1996, in part to legislation and education. The Minimum Drinking Age Laws have also helped reduce traffic fatalities in driver's age 18 to 20 by 13 percent. These laws have saved an estimated 14,586 lives between 1982–1998. (NHTSA, 1999)

As BAC increases, the likelihood of being involved in an alcohol related crash increases significantly. A driver with a BAC of .15 is more than 300 times more likely to be involved in a fatal crash (NHTSA, 1997). BAC levels as low as .02 affect driving ability and crash responsibility. The probability of a crash increases greatly at .05 BAC and begins a rapid increase at .08 BAC.

According to a 1999 published NHTSA report, in 1997 1.4 million people were arrested in the U.S. for DWI, and 21 percent of young drivers involved in fatal crashes had been drinking.

Although most drivers involved in fatal crashes have no prior convictions for DWI, about one third of all drivers arrested for DWI are repeat offenders, which greatly increases their risk of causing a drunk driving accident. In 1998, one out of nine intoxicated drivers in fatal crashes had a prior DWI conviction within the past three years (NHTSA, 1999).

Alcohol Use in College

The legal drinking age in all states is 21 years old but that does not mean individuals under 21 do not consume alcohol. In the U.S. in 1995, there were an estimated 10 million drinkers under the age of 21. Of these, 4.4 million were binge drinkers, including 1.7 million heavy drinkers (SAMHSA, 1996). Studies suggest that substance use, including alcohol, tobacco, and other drug use, is common among college-aged youth. Students who use any of these substances are at significantly greater risk than non-substance using peers to: drive after drinking and with a driver who has been drinking, and are less likely to use a seatbelt. These consistently poor and risky choices increase their risk of being in a motor vehicle crash and having crash-related injuries (Everett, 1999).

At campuses across the country, approximately 240,000 to 360,000 of the nation's 12 million undergraduates will die of an alcohol related cause (Eigen, 1991). College students who reported D/F GPAs consumed an average of 10 drinks per week while those who earned mostly As consumed slightly more than three drinks per week, if any at all (Core Institute, 1993). According to a 1995 report by the Center on Addiction and Substance Abuse at Columbia University:

- College students spend $5.5 billion dollars on alcohol per year, averaging $466/student/year.
- Alcohol is a factor in 40% of all academic problems and 28% of all dropouts
- In 90% of sexual assault cases, either the victim or the attacker was under the influence of alcohol
- 42% of students report that they had five drinks at one time in a two week period compared to 33% of their non-college counterparts
- 60 % of college women diagnosed with STDs were drunk at the time of infection

Binge Drinking

Binge drinking is defined as consuming five or more drinks at one sitting for men, and four or more for women. Binge drinkers usually experience more alcohol related problems than their

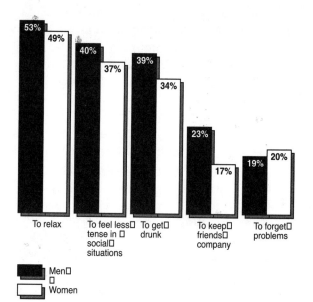

Adapted from Wechsler and McFadden for AAA foundation for Traffic Safety. Survey of 1669 college freshman at 14 Massachusetts institutions.

FIGURE 7.2 Why college freshmen drink. Survey respondents could choose more than one reason.

non-drinking counterparts (Harvard, 1997). These problems affect their health, education, safety and interpersonal relationships. According to the Harvard School of Public Health College Alcohol Study in 1997, these problems include driving after drinking, damaging property, getting injured, missing classes, and getting behind in school work. According to the same Harvard study, one in five students surveyed experienced five or more different alcohol-related problems and more than one-third of the students reported driving after drinking.

The study also found that the vast majority of non-binge drinking students are negatively affected by the behavior of binge drinkers. It was reported that four out of five students who were non-binge drinkers and who lived on campus experienced at least one effect of binge drinking such as being the victim of a sexual assault or an unwanted sexual advance, property vandalized, having sleep or study interrupted.

Drinking Problems

Nearly 14 million Americans, one in every 13 adults, abuse alcohol or are alcoholics. Rates of alcohol problems are highest among young adults ages 18–29 and lowest in adults ages 65 and older (NIAAA, 1995).

The National Institute on Alcohol Abuse and Alcoholism (NIAAA) found that the earlier young people begin to drink alcohol, the more likely they are to become an alcohol abuser or alcoholic. According to the report:

- Young people who start drinking before age 15 are four times more likely to become an alcoholic than if they start after age 21.
- 40 percent who drink before age 15 become alcohol dependant. 10 percent if they wait until 21.
- 14 percent decreased risk of alcoholism for each year drinking is delayed until age 21.

How Can You Tell if Someone Has a Drinking Problem?

There are many "red flags" that can point to a problem with alcohol. One way is to answer these questions developed by Dr. John Ewing:

- Have you ever felt you should CUT down on your drinking?
- Have people ANNOYED you by criticizing your drinking?
- Have you ever felt bad or GUILTY about your drinking?
- Have you ever had a drink first thing in the morning to steady your nerves or to get rid of the hangover (EYE OPENER)?

To help remember these questions, notice that the first letter of each key word spells CAGE. One "yes" answer suggests a possible alcohol problem. More than one "yes" means it is highly likely that a problem exists (Ewing, 1995).

Other signs and symptoms also could indicate that a person could be misusing or abusing alcohol or other drugs. One or two of them does not necessarily point to a problem, but several, combined with the right circumstances need to be addressed. Some of these signs may include a grade decline or a sudden drop in grades, frequently missing class because of hangovers, binge drinking, legal problems associated with alcohol or a significant increase in tolerance to alcohol. Other major signs of a drinking problem could be frequently drinking alone, drinking to forget about personal problems or avoiding activities where alcohol is not available. Another more serious physical sign of alcohol abuse is a *blackout*. This is when an individual has amnesia about events after drinking even though there was no loss of consciousness.

Alcoholism

Alcoholism, also known as alcohol dependence, is a chronic, progressive diseases with symptoms that include a strong need to drink and continue drinking despite repeated negative alcohol-related consequences. There are four symptoms generally associated with alcoholism: a craving or a strong need to drink, impaired control or the inability to limit one's drinking, a physical dependence accompanied by withdrawal symptoms such as nausea, sweating, shakiness and anxiety when alcohol use is stopped, and an increased tolerance.

Can Alcoholism Be Hereditary?

Alcoholism has a biological base. The tendency to become an alcoholic is inherited. Men and women are four times more likely to become alcoholics if their parents were (NIAAA, 1995). Currently researchers are finding the genes that influence vulnerability to alcohol. A person's environment may also play a role in drinking and the development of alcoholism. This is not destiny. A child of an alcoholic parent will not automatically develop alcoholism and a person with no family history of alcohol can become alcohol dependent.

There are ways to avoid becoming alcohol dependent. It is important to know your limit and stick to it. If choosing to drink, drink slowly and alternate an alcoholic beverage with a non-alcoholic beverage, eat while drinking, and most importantly find more effective ways of dealing with problems instead of turning to alcohol (Powell, 1996).

If you feel this is a problem, the sooner you stop, the better the chances of avoiding serious psychological effects.

- Admit to your drinking—first step in avoiding serious problems.
- Change your lifestyle—try to stay out of situations where alcohol is prominent until you can control your drinking.
- Get involved in self-help groups.

Alcohol Poisoning

Alcohol poisoning results when an overdose of alcohol is consumed. This is a medical emergency that requires immediate attention. Some symptoms of alcohol poisoning are:

- Person does not respond to talking, shouting, or being shaken
- Person cannot stand up
- Person has slow, labored, or abnormal breathing
- Person's skin feels clammy
- Person has a rapid pulse rate and irregular heart rhythm
- Person has lowered blood pressure

Choking to death on one's own vomit after an alcohol overdose is quite common. Death by asphyxiation occurs when alcohol depresses the body's reflexes to the point that the person cannot vomit properly.

What You Should Do:
- Call for medical attention immediately. Stay with the person until help arrives. **Do not leave the victim alone.**
- Turn the victim on to one side in case of vomiting.
- Be honest in telling medical staff exactly how much alcohol the victim consumed.

Chronic Effects

Drinking too much alcohol can cause a wide range of chronic health problems including liver disease, cancer, heart disease, nervous system problems as well as alcoholism. The Journal of the American Medical Association (JAMA), suggested that moderate levels of alcohol consumption (1-2 drinks per day) might reduce the risk of coronary heart disease (JAMA, 1994). However researchers report in a more recent issue of JAMA that moderate consumption of alcohol decreases the risk of stroke but heavy consumption increases the risk of stroke (JAMA, 1999). The National Stroke Association guidelines say that drinking one drink each day may actually lower the risk of stroke.

Although moderate amounts of alcohol may not be harmful, there are some major health issues associated with chronic alcohol use and abuse.

Liver disease is commonly associated with alcohol abuse. The liver has many vital functions in the body. It is a common mistake for people to think that only those individuals who abuse alcohol can harm the liver. Individuals who are heavy social drinkers may run the risk of liver damage as well.

Hepatotoxic trauma or "fatty liver" is the most common alcohol-related disorder causing enlargement of the liver. Some damage can be reversed if alcohol is completely avoided.

Alcoholic Hepatitis is an enlarged and tender liver with an elevation of white blood cells. Symptoms can include nausea, vomiting, abdominal pain, fever, and jaundice. If alcohol use continues, this could progress to cirrhosis.

Alcohol Cirrhosis results from continued alcohol use, this may cause permanent scar tissue to form when the liver cells are damaged. This problem usually occurs in ten to fifteen percent of people who consumed large quantities and can develop in as little as five years of heavy drinking.

Alcohol Pellagra is a deficiency of protein and niacin. Symptoms may include skin inflammation, gastro intestinal disorders, diarrhea, and mental and nervous disorders.

Malnutrition occurs from a lack of needed nutrients through prolonged alcohol consumption, by depressing the appetite and attacking the lining of the stomach. Heavy drinkers do not get the calories they need which triggers increased mineral loss and increases fatty acids because of the interference of the transfer of glucose into energy.

Polyneuritis is a condition caused by thyamin deficiency, which causes inflammation of several nerves and causes the drinker to become weak and have a tingling sensation.

Cancers—It is established that two to four percent of all cancer cases could be caused by alcohol use. Cancer of the upper digestive tract such as mouth, esophageal, pharynx and larynx can be attributed to alcohol use. Liver cancer as well as breast cancer may be caused by excessive alcohol consumption. Studies indicate that a woman's risk of developing breast cancer increases with age and alcohol consumption (JAMA, 1995).

Fetal Alcohol Syndrome—Alcohol crosses the placenta but experts don't know exactly how drinking causes problems for the fetus. It may directly affect the fetus or it may be acetaldehyde, the metabolic by-product of alcohol that is harmful to the fetus. Some researchers believe that alcohol effects on the placenta cause blood flow and nutrient deficiencies. Whatever the reason, drinking during pregnancy clearly puts infants at risk for birth defects (Herman, 1997).

Neurological Disorders Associated with Alcohol Use

Wernickes Disease is caused by a thiamine deficiency. Some symptoms include decreased mental functions, double vision, and involuntary oscillation of the eyeballs.

Korsakoff's Syndrome is caused by a B complex vitamin deficiency. Symptoms are amnesia, personality alterations and a loss of reality. This person may become apathetic and have difficulty walking.

Organizations

For information regarding alcohol use and abuse contact the National Institute on Alcohol Abuse and Alcoholism (NIAAA) or the National Council on Alcoholism (NCA). Both of these organizations provide information and support.

Alcoholics Anonymous (AA) is an organization designed to support and help individuals become sober and stay sober. AA has over 19,000 affiliated groups and more than 350,000 members across the U.S.

AA (212) 870-3400
http://www.alcoholic-anonymous.org

Al-Anon and *Alateen* are organizations designed to help family members of alcoholics to cope with problems.

800-344-2666
http://www.al-anon-alateen.org

Tobacco

Tobacco Components

The toxic components of tobacco include tar, nicotine, and carbon monoxide.

Tar is a by product of burning tobacco. Its composition is a dark, sticky substance that can be condensed from cigarette smoke. Tar contains many potent carcinogens and chemicals that irritate tissue in the lungs and promote chronic bronchitis and emphysema. These substances paralyze and destroy the cilia that line the bronchi causing "smoker's cough." Long-term exposure of extremely toxic tar to lung tissue can lead to the development of cancer.

Nicotine is a colorless, oily compound that is extremely poisonous in concentrated amounts. This highly addictive drug is a major contributor to heart and respiratory diseases causing short-term increases in blood pressure, heart rate and flow of

blood from the heart causing the arteries to narrow. A strong dependence on nicotine can occur after as little as three packs of cigarettes and is more addictive than cocaine or heroin. Because of its addictive effects, the Food and Drug Administration (FDA) has determined nicotine should be regulated.

At first, nicotine acts as a stimulant and then it tends to tranquilize the nervous system. The effects depend largely on how one chooses to smoke. Shallow puffs seem to increase alertness because low doses of nicotine facilitate the release of acetylcholine, which creates feelings of alertness. Long, deep drags tend to relax the smoker because high doses of nicotine block the flow of acetylcholine. Ninety percent of the nicotine inhaled while smoking is absorbed into the body, while 25–30 percent of nicotine is absorbed if the smoke is drawn only into the mouth, not the lungs.

Other side effects include inhibiting formation of urine, discoloration of the fingers, dulling the taste buds, and irritating the membranes in the mouth and throat. Because nicotine constricts blood vessels, it causes the skin to be clammy and have a pallid appearance, as well as reducing body temperature. Because of its highly addictive nature, withdrawal symptoms from nicotine can occur quite suddenly. These symptoms include irritability, anxiousness, hostility, food cravings, headaches, and the inability to concentrate.

Carbon Monoxide is an odorless, tasteless gas that is highly toxic. It reduces the amount of oxygen the blood can carry causing shortness of breath. Carbon monoxide ultimately damages the inner walls of the arteries, thus encouraging a build up of fat on the walls of the arteries, this is called atherosclerosis. Over time, this causes the arteries to narrow and harden, which may lead to a heart attack.

Approximately one percent of cigarette smoke and six percent of cigar smoke is carbon monoxide. It impairs normal function of the nervous system and is partially responsible for the increased risk of heart attacks and strokes in smokers.

Types of Tobacco Use

Smokeless Tobacco (Snuff, Chewing Tobacco)
With smokeless tobacco, one experiences the effects of nicotine without the exposure to tar and carbon monoxide. Particularly popular among

young adult males, approximately 22 million people use smokeless tobacco in the United States, approximately 2 million people under the age of 25 and nearly 20 percent of males in 9–12th grades. Of this 20 percent, one-third started at age 5, with the average starting at age 9 (Floyd, 1998).

The misconception about smokeless tobacco is that it is a safe alternative to cigarettes. This is actually not true. The nicotine in smokeless tobacco is about two to three times that of a cigarette, making it extremely addictive. It is absorbed through the mucous membranes of the mouth releasing cancer-causing nitrosamines and creating numerous problems. These problems include: bad breath, cardiovascular diseases, and decreased smelling and tasting abilities. Users tend to add more salt or sugar to food because of the decrease in taste ability, which can lead to hypertension and obesity. Dependency occurs because it is absorbed directly into the bloodstream from the mouth. This causes a dependency that is believed to be harder to break than smoking (Floyd, 1998).

Another major problem caused by smokeless tobacco is *leukoplakia*, which is a pre-cancerous condition that produces thick, rough, white patches on the gums, tongue, and inner cheeks. A variety of cancers such as lip, pharynx, larynx, esophagus, and tongue can be attributed to smokeless tobacco. Dental and gum problems are major side effects as well.

Cigarette Smoking

According to the American Heart Association, there are approximately 25.2 million male smokers in the United States, 23.2 million women, and 4.1 million teens between the ages of 12–17(AHA, 1999).

Cigarette smoking greatly impairs the respiratory system and is a major cause of Chronic Ob-

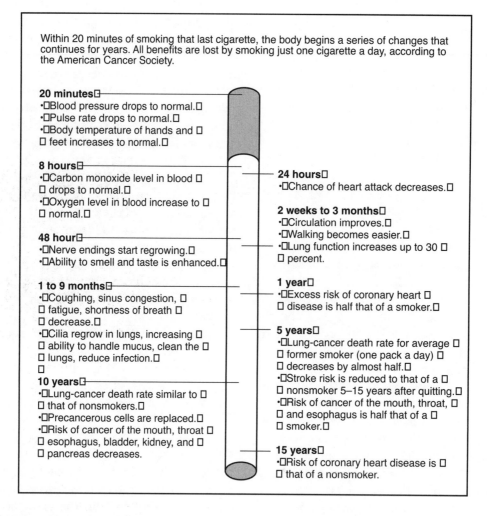

FIGURE 7.3 When smokers quit.

structive Pulmonary Diseases (COPD), which include emphysema and chronic bronchitis. The Surgeon General has stated that cigarette smoking is the largest preventable cause of illness and premature death in the United States. Smokers are ten times more likely to develop lung cancer than non-smokers. Fewer than 13 percent of smokers diagnosed with lung cancer survive for five years. Cigarette smokers are 20 times more likely to have heart attacks than non-smokers and smokers who smoke two packs a day are 15 to 25 times more likely to contract lung cancer than non-smokers (CDC, 1997). It has been estimated that each cigarette shortens your life by two minutes.

Problems associated with cigarette smoking include mouth, throat, and other types of cancer, cirrhosis of the liver, stomach and duodenal ulcers, gum and dental disease, decreased HDL cholesterol and decreased platelet survival and clotting time as well as increased blood thickness.

Cigarette smoking increases problems such as heart disease, atherosclerosis, blood clots, increases the amount of fatty acids, glucose, and various hormones in the blood, cardiac arrhythmia, allergies, diabetes, hypertension, peptic ulcers and sexual impotence.

Smoking doubles the risk of heart disease and smokers have only a fifty percent chance of recovery. Smokers also have a 70 percent higher death rate from heart disease than non-smokers (CDC, 1999). Smoking causes cardiomyopathy, which is a condition that weakens the heart's ability to pump blood.

Life expectancy of smokers parallels smoking habits in that the younger one starts smoking and the longer one smokes, the higher the mortality rate. Also, the deeper smoke is inhaled and the higher the tar and nicotine content, the higher the mortality rate.

Cigars/Other

The risk and mortality rates for lip, mouth, and larynx cancers for pipe and cigar smoking are higher than for cigarette smoking. Pipe smoke, which is 2% carbon monoxide, is more irritating to the respiratory system than cigarette smoking, but for those who do not inhale, the risk for developing cancer is just as likely.

Cigars have recently gained popularity in the U.S. among younger men and women with approximately 4.5 billion cigars consumed yearly.

Clove cigarettes are erroneously believed to be safer because they do not contain as much tobacco. In actuality, clove cigarettes are most harmful because they contain eugenol, which is an active ingredient of clove. Eugenol deadens sensations in the throat, which allow smokers to inhale more deeply and hold smoke in the lungs longer. Clove cigarettes also contain twice as much tar, nicotine, and carbon monoxide as most moderate brands of American cigarettes.

Environmental Tobacco Smoke

Environmental Tobacco Smoke, (ETS), which is also known as second hand smoke or passive smoke, reportedly causes 60,000 deaths each year. ETS may harm the cardiovascular system of non-smokers more than smokers and may increase the risk of non-fatal cardiac problems. Researchers have identified over 4,000 chemical compounds in tobacco, at least 43 of these compounds cause cancer in humans (CDC, 1999). The Environmental Protection Agency (EPA) officially declared ETS to be a human carcinogen in 1993. Each year because of exposure to ETS, an estimated 3,000 non-smoking Americans die of lung cancer and 12,000 a year die from other cancers. It is also estimated that 300,000 children suffer from lower respiratory tract infections. On the average, ETS triggers 23 asthma attacks every hour in children (CDC, 1999). As a result of these figures, in 1994 the Occupational Safety and Health Administration, OSHA, prohibited smoking in the workplace.

Statistical Information

The U.S. Surgeon General's Report in 1970 warned that cigarette smoking is dangerous to your health. The Surgeon General later describes cigarette smoking as "the number one preventable cause of death and health problems in our society." Each year smoking kills more people than alcohol, drugs, suicide, homicide, car accidents, fires and AIDS combined (CDC, 1998). The annual costs of smoking related problems are more than 50 billion dollars in direct medical costs.

Over 400,000 people die each year from smoking related problems. It is estimated that five million children living today will die prematurely because of a decision they will make as an adolescent, the decision to start smoking cigarettes (CDC, 1999).

According to a CDC report, in the 30 years since the first Surgeon General's Report on smoking:

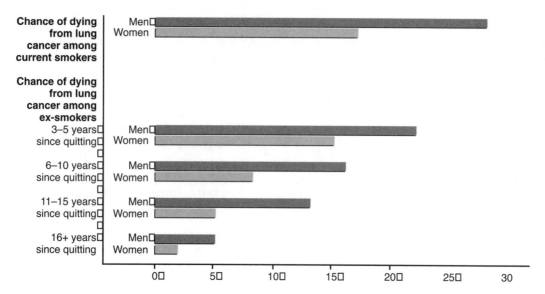

FIGURE 7.4 Lessened lung cancer risks. The 1990 U.S. Surgeon General's report concludes that smokers who quit significantly reduce their risks of dying from lung cancer.

Smoking and Health. (1990). Rockville, MD: Health and Human Services.

- Approximately 10 million people in the U.S. have died from a smoking-related cause
- More than 55 million people have started smoking
- American smokers have consumed 17 trillion cigarettes—if laid end to end, those cigarettes would cover 900 million miles
- American smokers have consumed approximately 300,000 tons of tar and 20,000 tons of nicotine

Women and Smoking

More than 145,000 women die every year from smoking related diseases. Lung cancer is the leading cause of death among women smokers (AHA, 1999). In addition to these statistics, women who smoke and take oral contraceptives, are 10 times more likely to have a heart attack than women who do neither.

Mothers who smoke during pregnancy are more likely to have low birth weight babies and put their babies at an increased risk of Sudden Infant Death Syndrome, SIDS. Dr. David Satcher in his first report as the Surgeon General in 1998, states that "not only does tobacco smoke shorten the lives of kids who start smoking but babies and children who are exposed to tobacco smoke have more ear infections, asthma, and a higher incidence of SIDS" (CDC, 1999).

Young People and Smoking

The Federal Office on Smoking and Health estimates that 3,000 young people begin smoking every day. According to the first report of the National Commission on Drug-free Schools, children and adolescents consume more than one billion packs of cigarettes a year. Economists estimate that the tobacco industry would need to recruit 5,000 new young smokers every day just to keep the constant total numbers of smokers—due to those who quit smoking or die.

The Department of Health and Human Services states that 90 percent of smokers begin tobacco use before age 20, and 50 percent begin tobacco use by age 14, with 25 percent beginning their addiction by age 12 (AHA, 1998).

It is because of these staggering statistics that the tobacco industry targets young people with their advertisements. For example, the Joe Camel ads by R. J. Reynolds Tobacco Company which have been recently terminated, offered many promotional items that are very appealing to young people. Neon camel signs, leather jackets, sandals all in exchange for coupons. A person would have to smoke up to 600 packs of Camels to receive some of the items (AHA, 1999).

Smoking Cessation

Each year an estimated 1.3 million smokers quit successfully, more than four out of five smokers say they want to quit (AHA, 1999).

Although there are various pharmacological agents used to aid smokers in quitting, nicotine replacement therapy has been shown to be the most effective. The transdermal nicotine patch is safe as well as nicotine gum, though the patch appears to be preferred by most. In addition to the patch and gum, a nicotine nasal spray and nicotine inhalers are also available.

Of the 48 million Americans who currently smoke cigarettes, most are either actively trying to quit or want to quit (AHA, 1999). Since 1965, more than 40% of all adults who have ever smoked have quit.

Quitting can bring a major reduction in the occurrence of coronary heart disease and other forms of cardiovascular diseases. Quitting reduces the risk for repeat heart attacks and death from heart disease by 50 percent or more (AHA, 1999). Quitting can also aid in the management of contributors to heart attacks such as, atherosclerosis, thrombosis and cardiac arrhythmia. 25 percent of the adult population smokes, which is considerably down from the 42 percent in 1965.

By choosing to quit smoking, the American Heart Association reports that after one year off cigarettes, risk for heart attacks is reduced by 50 percent. After 15 years of abstinence from smoking your risks are similar to that of a person whom never smoked. In five to 15 years of being smoke-free, the risk of stroke is the same as for non-smokers. Male smokers who quit between ages 35–39 add an average of five years to their lives, and females add three years to their lives (AHA, 1999).

There is some irreversible damage to virtually every organ system in the body. There are dangers from smoking that remain even after quitting. Although it is never too late to quit smoking, the damage that has been done may never entirely disappear. It is better to choose to never light up!

Contacts

American Council on Science and Health(ACSH)
1995 Broadway, 2nd Floor
New York, NY 10023-5860
(212)362-7044
http://www.acsh.org

American Heart Association(AHA)
National Center
7272 Greenville Avenue
Dallas, TX 75231
1-800-AHA-USA1
http://www.aha.org

American Lung Association(ALA)
1740 Broadway
New York, NY 10019-4274
(212)315-8700
1-800-LUNG-USA
http://www.lungusa.org/
American Medical Association (AMA)
515 North State Street
Chicago, IL 60610
(312)464-5000
http://www.ama-assn.org/

Centers for Disease Control and Prevention
http://www.cdc.gov/tobacco

U.S. Department of Health and Human Services
Action on Smoking and Health (ASH)
2013 H Street, N.W.
Washington, D.C. 20006
(202)659-4310
http://ash.org

The Advocacy Institute (AI)
1707 L Street, N.W.
Washington, D.C. 20036-4505
(202)659-8475
http://www.advocacy.org/tobacco.htm

American Cancer Society (ACS)
1599 Clifton Road, N.E.
Atlanta, Ga 30329
1-800-ACS-2345
http://www.cancer.org

Americans for Nonsmoker's Rights (ANR)
Suite J
2530 San Pablo Avenue
Berkley, CA 94702
(510)841-3032
http://www.no-smoke.org/

Association of State and Territorial Health Officials (ASTHO)
1275 K Street, NW
Suite 800
Washington, DC 20005
(202)371-9090
http://www.astho.org/

Cancer Research Foundation of America (CRFA)
1600 Duke Street
Alexandria, VA 22314
(703)836-4412
http://www.preventcancer.org

Doctors Ought to Care (DOC)
5615 Kirby Drive
Suite 440
Houston, TX 77005
(713)528-1487
http://www.bcm.tmc.edu/doc/

Psychoactive Drugs

It is estimated that one in five females and one in three males abuses drugs or becomes addicted to drugs at some time in his or her life (Floyd, 1998). According to the National Center on Addiction and Substance Abuse at Columbia University, the highest rate for illegal drug use is among the 18–25 year-old age group. People choose to take drugs for many reasons. Some choose to experiment while others try to escape from reality. Whatever the reason, the effects can be deadly.

Psychoactive drugs are classified into six categories according to their physiological effects on the body: stimulants, depressants, hallucinogens, cannabis, narcotics, and inhalants. All psychoactive drugs serve to disrupt the normal functioning of the central nervous system. By interrupting the transfer of electrical impulses from neurotransmitters (chemical messengers) across the synapses between nerve cells (dendrites). Several different changes to the neurotransmitters may occur depending on the drug. The deactivation of the impulse may not occur thus allowing for continuous stimulation, or the drug may allow for a continuous slow release of the neurotransmitter. An altered neurotransmitter can result from psychoactive drug use or the stimuli could be totally blocked. Neurotransmitters are important to the relay of information within this system. Substances that interrupt neurotransmitter function seriously disrupt the function of the nervous system.

Types of Drugs

Stimulants

Amphetamines are drugs that speed up the nervous system. They do not occur naturally and must be manufactured in a laboratory. When used in moderation, amphetamines stimulate receptor sites for two naturally occurring neurotransmitters, having the effect of elevated moods, increased alertness, and feelings of well being. In addition, the activity of the stomach and intestines may be slowed and appetite suppressed. When amphetamines are eliminated from the body, the user becomes fatigued. With abuse, the user will experience rapid tolerance and a strong psychological dependence, along with the possibility of impotence and episodes of psychosis. When use stops, the abuser may experience periods of depression.

The most commonly abused amphetamine today is *methamphetamine*, commonly called "crank," "ice," "crystal," "meth," "speed," "crystal meth," and "zip." The most dangerous form of methamphetamine is crystal methamphetamine, which looks like rock candy. This is smoked rather than ingested. The effects of this drug are rapid and can last for several hours, leaving the user physically exhausted. The increase in this drug's popularity has resulted in reports of violence, psychotic behavior, and homicide. Long term abuse can result in nutritional difficulties, weight loss, reduced resistance to infections and damage to the liver, lungs, and kidneys.

Cocaine is a naturally occurring psychoactive substance contained in the leaves of the South American coca plant. Crack cocaine, a rock-like crystalline form of cocaine made by combining cocaine hydrochloride with common baking soda, can be heated in the bowl of a pipe enabling the vapors to be inhaled into the lungs. Cocaine is used occasionally as a topical anesthetic medicinally, however, more commonly it is inhaled (snorted), injected, or smoked illegally. The effects of cocaine use are rapid and short lived (from 5 to 30 minutes). Snorting enables only about 60 percent of the drug to be absorbed because the nasal vessels constrict immediately. Cocaine use causes dopamine and norepinephrine to be released into the brain causing a feeling of euphoria and confidence, however, at the same time electrical impulses to the heart that regulate its rhythm are impaired. There is evidence that both psychological and physical dependence on cocaine occur rapidly.

TABLE 7.1. Common Sources of Caffeine

	Milligrams		Milligrams
Coffee (6-oz. cup)		Tea (6-oz. cup)	
Brewed, drip method	80–175	Brewed	53
Decaffeinated, brewed	3	Instant	30
Instant	60–100	Oolong	36
Decaffeinated, instant	2	Green	32
Espresso (2 oz.)	90–120	Analgesics	
Chocolate		Actamin Super, Aspirin-free	
Dark chocolate (1 oz.)	5–35	Excedrin, Excedrin Extra	
Chocolate cake (1 slice)	20–30	Strength	65
Milk chocolate (1 oz.)	1–10	Goody's Headache Powders,	
Chocolate-flavored syrup (1 oz.)	4	Supac, Vanquish	33
Soft drinks (12 oz.)		Anacin, Anacin Maximum	
Jolt Cola	72	Strength, Buffets II, Cope, Gelprin,	
Sundrop	63	Gensan, P-A-C Revised formula,	
Kick	58	Rid-A-Pain Compound, Midol	32
Mountain Dew	55	Cold-allergy remedies	
Mellow Yellow	52	Kolephrin, Kolephrin/DM	65
Coca-Cola	47	Fendol	32
Diet Coke	47	Triaminicin, Histosal	30
Mr. Pibb	41	Dristan AF Decongestant	16
Dr. Pepper	41	Stimulants	
Sunkist Orange	40	Caffedrine, Keep Alert, NoDoz Maximum	
Pepsi-Cola	38	Strength, Ultra Pep-Back, Vivarin	200
Diet Pepsi	36	Quick Pep	150
A & W Cream Soda	28	NoDoz, Pep-Back	100
Barq's	23	Enerjets	75
Slice Cola	11	Weight Control	
Water, caffeine enhanced (12 oz.)		Dexatrim Extra Strength	200
Java Water	71	Diuretics	
Krank $_2$O	70	Permathene H$_2$ Off	200
Water Joe	46	Aqua-Ban	100
Aqua Java	43		
Juice drinks, caffeine enhanced (12 oz.)			
Java Juice	90		
XTC	70		

Data on coffee, tea, tea products, and chocolate products: Institute of Food Technologists. (1987, June). Evaluation of Caffeine Safety. Data on soft drinks: National Soft Drink Association.

Today, the smoking of crack cocaine is more prevalent than inhalation. When smoked, the drug reaches the central nervous system immediately, effecting several neurotransmitters in the brain. The effects are short lived (usually around 5-10 minutes) leaving the user with feelings of depression. Abuse of this drug can result in convulsions, seizures, respiratory distress, and sudden cardiac failure.

The relatively short lived "high" from cocaine requires frequent use to maintain feelings of euphoria and is therefore quite costly for the addict. A single dose of crack sells for $30 or more, so to maintain a habit would cost hundreds of dollars a day. To pay for their habit, addicts will often turn to criminal activities such as dealing drugs, stealing, or prostitution. Crack houses are known for promoting the spread of HIV infection and thousands of babies are born to crack-addicted mothers. These babies have severe physical and neurological problems, requiring significant medical attention. The cost of this drug is high, not just for the user, but for society as well.

Caffeine is a stimulant as well as a psychotropic (mind affecting) drug. Caffeine is generally associated with coffee, tea, and cola, but can also be found in chocolate, cocoa, and other carbonated beverages, as well as some medications, both prescription and non-prescription, i.e. Excedrin®. Approximately 65-180 milligrams of caffeine are found in one cup of coffee, compared to tea, which contains 40-100 milligrams per cup and cola which contains 30-60 milligrams per 12 ounce can. Caffeine is readily absorbed into the body and causes stimulation of the cerebral cortex and medullary centers in the brain, resulting in mental alertness.

"Normal consumption" of caffeine, as little as 75-200 milligrams per day may quicken reaction time, masks fatigue, relieves drowsiness, and may help in performance of repetitive tasks. It also acts as a diuretic and can stimulate gastric secretions.

Excessive consumption of caffeine increases plasma levels of epinephrine, norepinephrine and renin. It also can cause serious side effects, such as tremors, nervousness, irritability, headaches, hyperactivity, arrhythmia, dizziness, and insomnia. It can elevate the blood pressure and body temperature, increase the breathing rate, irritate the stomach and bowels, and dehydrate the body. Excessive amounts of caffeine may increase the incidence of Premenstrual Syndrome (PMS) in some women and may increase fibrocystic breast disease (non-cancerous breast lumps) as well. The U.S. Surgeon General recommends that women avoid or restrict caffeine intake during pregnancy. Withdrawal symptoms from caffeine may include headaches, depression, drowsiness, nervousness, and a feeling of lethargy.

Depressants

Depressants are sedatives or anxiolytic (anti-anxiety) drugs that depress the central nervous system, reducing or relieving tension and/or anxiety, and inducing relaxation, drowsiness, or sleep.

Benzodiazepines, the most widely used group of depressants are prescribed to relieve tension, muscle strain, sleep disturbances, panic attacks, anesthesia, or treatment for alcohol withdrawal and sometimes used to treat epileptic seizures. Examples include Librium, Valium, Serax, Ativan, Dalmand, and Xanax. All of these differ in action, absorption, and metabolism, but all produce similar intoxication and withdrawal symptoms.

Barbiturates are used to induce relaxation, sleep and relieve tension. They are usually taken orally in tablet, capsule, or liquid form, but when used as a general anesthetic, taken intravenously, they work as a serious respiratory depressant.

There are two types of barbiturates, short acting and long acting. The short acting barbiturate are rapidly absorbed into the brain. Examples are Nembutal ("Yellow Jackets"), Secobarbital—Seconal ("Reds"), and Thiopental (Pentothal). Long acting barbiturates are taken orally and absorbed slowly into the bloodstream, lasting for several days. Examples are Amobarbital (Amytal—"blues," or "downers"), and Phenobarbital (Luminal—"phennies").

Depressants can produce both a physical and psychological dependence within two to four weeks. Those with a prior history of abuse are at greater risk of abusing sedatives, even if prescribed by a physician. If there is no previous substance abuse history, one rarely develops problems if prescribed and monitored by a physician. Depressants can be very dangerous, if not lethal, if used in combination with alcohol, leading to respiratory depression, respiratory arrest, and death.

Cross-tolerance is a specific complication with sedatives. A person who is addicted to one sedative will likely develop a tolerance for other sedatives as well.

Some of the physiological effects of depressants include drowsiness, impaired judgement, poor coordination, slowed breathing, confusion, weak and rapid heartbeat, relaxed muscles and pain relief.

A major health risk associated with the use of depressants is the development of a dependence to the drug, leading to serious side effects, such as stupors, coma, and death. The withdrawal symptoms from depressant use can cause fatal reactions as well. Symptoms can range from relatively mild discomfort to severe discomfort (with grand mal seizures), depending on the degree of dependence. Withdrawal symptoms can begin two to three days after stopping drug use and persist for several weeks. Individuals who have developed a dependency on depressants should seek medical attention when trying to quit or decrease the dosage.

Narcotics

Narcotics are drugs that relieve pain and often induce sleep. Opium, derived from poppy seeds, is the base compound used for all narcotics. Opiates, which are narcotics, include opium and other drugs derived from opium, such as morphine, codeine, and heroin. Methadone is a synthetic chemical that has a morphine-like action, and also falls into this category of drugs.

Morphine is the main alkaloid found in opium. It is ten times stronger than opium and brings quick relief from pain. It is most effectively used as an anesthetic during heart surgery, to relieve pain in post operative patients, and some times used to relieve pain for cancer patients

Codeine is a natural derivative of opium, medically used as a mild painkiller or a cough suppressant. Although widely used, there is potential for physical dependence.

Heroin is considered a semi synthetic narcotic because it is derived from a naturally occurring substance in the Oriental poppy plant called opium. It is a highly effective, fast acting analgesic (painkiller) if injected when used medicinally; however, its benefits are outweighed by its risk of toxicity and high dependence rate. When injected or "skin popped" (injected beneath the skin's surface), a dream-like euphoria is produced. Abuse is common because this drug creates a strong physical and psychological dependence and tolerance. Recently heroin has become more popular among young people. The risks of heroin use are increased

due to the use of needles for injection. There is an increased likelihood of transmission of communicable diseases like HIV due to the practice of sharing needles. Although abrupt withdrawal from heroin is rarely fatal, the discomfort associated with going "cold turkey" is extremely intense.

Heroin accounts for 90 percent of the narcotic abuse in the U.S. Anyone can become dependant and life expectancy of the heroin addict who ingests the drug intravenously is significantly lower than that of one who does not. Overdose of heroin can result in death within minutes.

Withdrawal symptoms occur within 4-6 hours after the last injection. Full blown withdrawal symptoms such as shaking, sweating, vomiting, muscle aches, abdominal pains, and diarrhea, may begin within 12-16 hours of last injection. The intensity of these symptoms is relative to the severity of the addiction.

Cannabis

Marijuana is a naturally occurring plant called *Cannabis sativa*, whose leaves and stems can be dried, crushed and the mixture rolled in cigarettes (joints) and smoked. The fibers of this plant are also used to manufacture hemp rope and paper. The resins scraped from the flowering tops of the plant yield hashish, a form of marijuana that can be smoked in a pipe. The amount of the active ingredient, Tertahydrocannabinol (THC), determines the potency of the hallucinogenic affect. Because THC is a fat-soluable substance, it is absorbed and retained in the fat tissues of the body for up to a month. Drug tests can detect trace amounts of THC for up to three weeks after consumption. Medicinal uses include relief of the nausea caused by chemotherapy, improvement of appetite in AIDS patients, and the relief of pressure in the eyes of glaucoma patients. The effects of marijuana use vary from user to user, but usually result in some similar experiences. Users report food cravings, a relaxed mood, and a heightened sensitivity to music. The behavioral effects on users include an impairment of short-term memory, an overestimation of the passage of time, and loss of ability to maintain attention to a task.

The long-term effects are still being studied, however, chronic abuse may lead to a motivational syndrome in some. Marijuana smoke is irritating to the lung tissues and may be more damaging than cigarette smoke. There are 400 chemicals in marijuana linked to lung cancer development. In addition, the immune system and reproductive systems are damaged. There is an increase in birth defects in mothers who smoke marijuana. The drug distorts perception and therefore is very dangerous when used while driving. The biggest concern related to marijuana use is the perception that there is no risk or harm associated with occasional use.

Hallucinogens

Hallucinogens, also called psychedelics, are drugs which affect perception, sensation, awareness and emotion. Changes in time and space and hallucinations may be mild or extreme depending on the dose, and may vary on every occasion. There are many synthetic as well as natural hallucinogens in use. Synthetic groups include LSD, which is the most potent, Mescaline, which is derived from the peyote cactus and psilocybin, derived from mushrooms, have similar effects.

LSD is a colorless, odorless and tasteless liquid that is made from lysergic acid which come from the ergot fungus. It was first converted to *lysergic acid diethylamide* (LSD) in 1938. In 1943, its psychoactive properties accidentally became known (SADA, 1999).

Hallucinations and illusions often occur, and effects vary according to the dosage, personality of the user and condition under which the drug is used. A flashback is a recurrence of some hallucinations from previous LSD experience days or months after the dose. Flashbacks can occur without reason, occurring to heavy users more frequently. After taking LSD, a person loses control over normal thought process. Street LSD is often mixed with other substances and its effects are quite uncertain.

Phencyclidine hydrochloride, also known as PCP or angel dust, is sometimes considered a hallucinogen although it does not easily fit into any category. First synthesized in 1959, it is used intravenously and as an anesthetic that blocks pain without producing numbness. Taken in small doses, it causes feelings of euphoria. It's harmful side effects include depression, anxiety, confusion, and delirium.

High doses of PCP cause mental confusion and hallucinations and can cause serious mental illness and extreme aggressive and violent behavior, including murder.

Inhalants

Inhalants are chemicals that produce vapors having psychoactive effects when sniffed. Inhalants are considered delerients which can damage the heart, brain, lungs, and liver. Common inhalants include model glue, acetone, gasoline, kerosene, nail polish, aerosol sprays, Pam™ cooking spray, Scotchgard™ fabric protectant, lighter fluids, butane, and cleaning fluids as well as nitrous oxide (laughing gas).

Inhalants reach the lungs, bloodstream, and other parts of the body very quickly. Intoxication can occur in as little as five minutes and can last as long as nine hours. Inhaled lighter fluid/butane displaces the oxygen in the lungs causing suffocation. Even a single episode can cause asphyxiation or cardiac arrhythmia and possibly leading to death.

The initial effects of inhalants are similar to those of alcohol, but they are very unpredictable. Some effects include, dizziness and blurred vision, involuntary eye movement, poor coordination, involuntary extremity movement, slurred speech, euphoric feeling, nose bleeds, and possible coma.

Health risks involved with the use of inhalants may include hepatitis, liver and/or kidney failure, as well as the destruction of bone marrow and skeletal muscles. Respiratory impairment and blood abnormalities, along with irregular heart beat and/or heart failure are also serious side effects of inhalants. Regular use can lead to tolerance and the need for more powerful drugs.

Some specific signs of inhalant abuse can be a rash around the nose and mouth, nosebleeds, residue found on the face, hands, or clothing, as well as breath odors. Redness, tearing or swelling of the eyes, irritation of the throat, lungs, and nose that may lead to gagging and coughing are also considered signs of inhalant abuse.

Other abused drugs

Ecstasy

MDMA or Ecstasy is chemically similar to methamphetamines and mescaline and has hallucinogenic effects. It is usually taken orally, but can be injected or inhaled and causes panic, anxiety, and rapid heart rate. An overdose can be lethal, especially when taken with alcohol or other drugs, i.e. heroin (H-bomb).

Rohypnol

Rohypnol (Flunitrazepam) is an illegal drug in the U.S., but an approved medicine in other parts of the world, where it is generally prescribed for sleep disorders. A 2 milligram tablet is equal to the potency of a six pack of beer. Rohypnol is a tranquilizer, similar to Valium, but 10 times more potent, producing sedative effects including muscle relaxation, dizziness, memory loss and blackouts. The effects occur 20–30 minutes after use and lasts for up to eight hours.

Rohypnol, more commonly known as "roofies," is a small, white, tasteless, pill that dissolves in food or drinks. It is most commonly used with other drugs, such as alcohol, Ecstasy, heroin, and marijuana to enhance the feeling of the other drug. Although Rohypnol alone can be very dangerous, as well as physically addicting, when mixed with other drugs, it can be fatal. It is also referred to as the "Date Rape" drug because there have been many reported cases of individuals giving Rohypnol to someone without their knowledge. Because the effects can be so severe, the individual is unaware he or she has been drugged and therefore is unable to resist an attack.

Gamma Hydroxybutyrate,
Gamma Hydroxybutyrate, GHB, is a fast-acting powerful drug that depresses the nervous system. GHB occurs naturally in the body in small amounts. First synthesized in the 1960s, GHB was once sold in health food stores as a performance-enhancing additive in body building supplements.

Commonly taken with alcohol, it depresses the central nervous system and induces an intoxicated state. GHB is commonly consumed orally, usually as a clear liquid or a white powder. It is odorless, colorless, and slightly salty to taste. Effects from GHB can occur within 15–30 minutes. Small doses (less than 1 gram) of GHB act as a relaxant with larger doses causing strong feelings of relaxation and slow heart rate and respiration. There is a very fine line to cross to a lethal dose which can lead to seizures, respiratory distress, low blood pressure and coma.

According to the Drug Abuse Warning Network, The Drug Induced Rape Prevention and Punishment Act of 1996 was enacted into federal law in response to the abuse of Rohypnol and GHB. This law makes it a crime to give someone a controlled substance without his/her knowledge and with the intent to commit a crime. The law also stiffens the penalties for possession and distribution of Rohypnol and GHB.

Used in Europe as a general anesthetic and treatment for insomnia, GHB is growing in popularity and is widely available under ground, manufactured by non-professional "kitchen" chemists, concerns about quality and purity should be considered.

Anabolic Steroids
There are two types of steroids in the body. Anabolic steroids build tissue and catabolic steroids break down or block processes. Catabolic are frequently used to treat arthritis, certain cancers and some skeletal disorders.

Anabolic steroids are synthetic male hormones or androgens. The term anabolic means these steroids affect tissue growth in the body. Side effects diminish the normal production of testosterone.

Steroid use can cause liver problems, kidney disease, shrinking testicles, sterility, high blood pressure, acne, sleep disorders and heart disease. Many users experience increased aggressive behavior, extreme mood swings, and depression. Sharing needles, suicide, and violent behavior are a few of the serious side effects associated with steroid use (Monaco, 1999).

References

Alcohol Alert. National Institute on Alcohol Abuse and Alcoholism, No.15, PH 311, January, 1992. No. 21, PH 345, July, 1993. No.31, PH 362, January 1996, Bethesda, MD.

Alcohol, Vision and Driving. American Automobile Association. Falls Church, VA, 1994.

American Heart Association. Annual Report, 1999.

Bain, et al. Diet and Melanoma: An Exploratory Case-Control Study. *Annual of Epidemiology*, Vol 3, No. 3, 1993.

Blomberg, Richard D. Lower BAC Limits for Youth: Evaluation of the Maryland .02 Law. DOT HS 807860, NHTSA, March, 1992, p. 17.

Commission on Substances Abuse at Colleges and Universities. Center on Addiction and Substance Abuse at Columbia University (CASA), 1994.

"College and University Students: Youth and Alcohol" Selected Reports to the Surgeon General, U.S. Department of Education (1993) PH-334.

Dennis, Maurice E. and The Texas Commission on Alcohol and Drug Abuse. *Instructor Manual, Alcohol Education Program for Minors.* TCADA, 1998.

Eigen, Lewis. "Alcohol Practices, Policies and Potentials of American Colleges and Universities," Department of Health and Human Services, 1991.

Everett, Sherry A., et al. "Unsafe Motor Vehicle Practices among Substance Using College Students." *Accident Analysis and Prevention.* 1999.

Ewing, J.A. "Detecting Alcoholism: The CAGE Questionnaire." *Journal of American Medical Association.* 252 (14): 1905-1907, 1984.

Facts and Figures on College Youth. NCADI.

Floyd, Patricia A. *Personal Health: Perspectives and Lifestyles,* 2d ed. Englewood, CO: Morton Publishing, 1998.

Hales, Dianne. *An Invitation to Health.* 8th ed. New York: Brooks/Cole Publishing Company, 1999.

Harvard School of Public Health College Alcohol Study, 1997.

Herman, Journal of the American Medical Association, 1997.

Hoeger, Werner and Sharon Hoeger. *Principle and Labs for Fitness and Wellness.* 5th ed., Englewood, CO: Morton Publishing Company, 1999.

Hot Issues: Binge Drinking on Campuses *Join Together,* http://www.jointogether.org.

Hot Issues: Binge Drinking on Campuses: The Fact Is. distributed by *Join Together.* http://www.jointogether.org.

Journal of American Medical Association, 1994 and 1999.

Jensen, R. Juvenile and Family Court Journal, 33:4, 1998, pp. 63-66.

Kenney, J. and G. Leaton. *Loosening the Grip.* 5th ed. St. Louis, MO: Mosby Publishing, 1995.

Longnecker. Alcoholic Beverage Consumption in Relation to Risk of Breast Cancer: Meta-Analysis and Review. *Cancer Causes and Control,* Vol. 5, 1994.

Maisto, Stephen, et al. *Drug Use and Abuse.* 2d ed. Fort Worth, Tx: The Hardcourt Press, 1995.

Making the Link: Violence and Crime and Alcohol and Other Drugs. Center for Substance Abuse Protection.

Martin, Susan. The Epidemiology of Alcohol Related Interpersonal Violence. *Alcohol Health and Research.* 18:3, 1994.

Mayhew, M.A. and H.M. Simpson. Alcohol, Age, and Risk of Road Accident Involvement.

Alcohol, Drugs, and Traffic Safety. Proceedings of the 9th International Conference on Alcohol, Drugs, and Traffic Safety, 1983, pp. 937-947.

National Highway Traffic Safety Administration, Fatal Accident Reporting System, 1998.

National Institute on Drug Abuse, *www.nida.nih.gov.*

National Institute on Alcohol Abuse and Alcoholism, 1995 and 1995.

O'Malley, P.M. and A.C. Wagenaar. Effects of Minimum Drinking Age Laws and Traffic Crash Involvement Among American Youth: 1976-1987. *Journal of Studies on Alcohol,* 52: 5, 1991.

Payne, Wayne A. and Hahn, Dale P. *Understanding Your Health.* New York: WCB McGraw-Hill, 1995.

Prentice, William E. *Fitness and Wellness for Life,* 6th ed. New York: WCB McGraw-Hill, 1999.

Powell. National Institute on Alcohol Abuse and Alcoholism, 1995.

Ray, Oakley and Ksir Charles. *Drugs, Society and Human Behavior.* 8th ed. St. Louis: Times Mirror/Mosby College Publishing 1999.

Robbins, Gwen, Debbie Powers, and Sharon Burgess. *A Wellness Way of Life.* 4th ed. New York: WCB McGraw-Hill, 1999.

Significant Developments Related to Smoking and Health. 1997. Centers for Disease Control and Prevention.

Students Against Drug Abuse. http://www.sada.org.

Substance Abuse and Mental Health Services Administration, SAMHSA, National Clearinghouse for Alcohol and Drug Abuse, http://www.samhsa.gov.

Texas Department of Public Safety. Motor Vehicle Traffic Accidents. Department of Public Safety, Austin, Texas, 1996.

U.S. Department of Health and Human Services, Centers for Disease Control and Prevention Annual Report, 1999. http://www.cdc.gov

Web of Addictions. http://www.well.com/user/woa.

Women and Alcohol: Use and Abuse. Author unknown. *The Journal of Nervous and Mental Disease.* 181: 4, Serial Number 1325, April, 1993.

Notebook Activities

Are You Addicted to Nicotine?

What Kind of Drinker Are You?

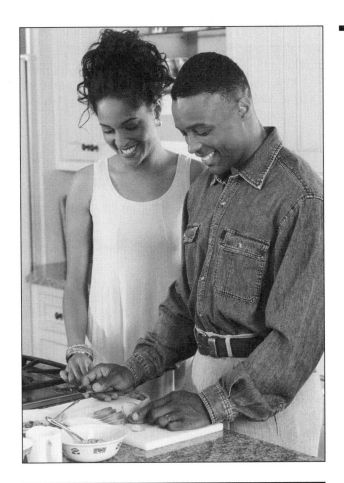

Chapter Eight

Nutrition

"A man's health can be judged by which he takes two at a time—pills or stairs."

—Joan Welsh

OBJECTIVES

Students will be able to:

- define the essential nutrients (carbohydrates, fats, proteins, vitamins, and minerals) and describe their roles in daily nutrition.

- introduce and explain the USDA Food Guide Pyramid.

- introduce guidelines for food labeling and explain how food labels describe the nutritional values of food.

- identify problems associated with fast food dining.

- discuss diet supplements.

- define the four styles of vegetarians.

- present guidelines for a successful weight-loss program.

- define eating disorders: who is at risk, what are the causes, what are the symptoms, how serious are they, and what can be done to help someone with an eating disorder.

Good, sound nutritional practices are necessary for maintaining a healthy lifestyle. Making an effort to obtain the essential nutrients through daily dietary intake is not something at which most Americans are proficient. In general, Americans eat too much salt, sugar, and fat, and do not consume the recommended daily allowance (RDA) of vitamins and minerals.

Poor dietary habits have been proven to contribute to the prevalence of diseases such as cardiovascular disease, obesity, and certain types of cancer. With this in mind, the importance of developing a knowledge base that will allow an individual to develop sound, lifelong nutritional practices becomes clear.

Once an individual has gathered the information that will allow them to make good nutritional choices, that person must then make a concentrated effort to obtain essential macronutrients and micronutrients through their daily dietary intake. *Macronutrients* provide energy in the form of calories, and they include carbohydrates, fats, and proteins. *Micronutrients,* which include vitamins and minerals, regulate many bodily functions such as, metabolism, growth, and development. Together, macronutrients and micronutrients are responsible for the following three tasks which are necessary for the continuance of life: 1) growth, repair, and maintenance of all tissues, 2) regulation of body process, and 3) providing energy.

Because nutrition information can often be misleading and appear overly complicated, several government agencies have published materials in an effort to decrease the amount of misinforma- tion available on nutrition, and increase the preva- lence of practical, applicable, "real world" infor- mation.

In 1995, the United Stated Department of Agri- culture and the Department of Health and Human Services published a revision of the Dietary Guide- lines for Americans. These seven guidelines, dis- played in Table 8.1, can serve as the basis of a nutritious and healthy diet.

TABLE 8.1. The 1995 Dietary Guidelines for Americans

1. **Eat a variety of foods.**
   No one food contains all the nutrients in the amounts needed. These nutrients should come from a variety of foods, not from a few highly fortified foods or supplements. Choose the rec- ommended number of servings from each of the five major food groups in the Food Guide Pyramid. Also select a variety of foods within each group. The content of your diet over a day or more is what counts!

2. **Balance the food you eat with physical activity—maintain or improve your weight.**
   Many Americans gain weight in adulthood, increasing their risk for high blood pressure, heart disease, diabetes, certain types of cancer, and other illnesses. Therefore, most adults should not gain weight, especially in the abdominal area (where excess fat is most dangerous). Most Americans spend much of their working day in activities that require little energy; try to do 30 minutes or more of moderate physical activity on most days of the week. Healthy low-fat eat- ing and exercise habits can help reduce health risks.

3. **Choose a diet with plenty of grain products, vegetables, and fruits.**
   These foods provide complex carbohydrates, dietary fiber, and other components linked to good health. These foods are also generally low in fat. The antioxidant nutrients in plant foods are potentially beneficial in reducing the risk for cancer.

4. **Choose a diet low in fat, saturated fat, and cholesterol.**
   Diets high in fat and cholesterol have been linked to heart disease, certain types of cancer, and obesity. Thirty percent or less of calories should come from fat, with less than 10 percent of calories from saturated fat. All adults are advised to have blood cholesterol levels checked.

5. **Choose a diet moderate in sugars.**
   Sugars and many foods that contain large amount of them supply calories but are limited in nu- trients. They also contribute to tooth decay.

6. **Choose a diet moderate in salt and sodium.**
   Most Americans eat more salt and sodium than they need, and using less will benefit those peo- ple whose blood pressure goes up with salt intake. Foods and beverages containing salt pro- vide most of the sodium in our diets, much of it added during processing and manufacturing.

7. **If you drink alcoholic beverages, do so in moderation.**
   Alcoholic beverages supply calories but few or no nutrients. The alcohol in these beverages has ef- fects that are harmful when the beverages are consumed in excess. These effects include altered judgment, potential dependency, and a great many other serious health problems.

---

*Recommendations for healthy Americans age 2 years and over.

Source: U.S. Department of Agriculture, U.S. Department of Health and Human Services. "Nutrition and Your Health: Dietary Guidelines for Americans," 4th ed. *Home and Garden Bulletin* no. 232 (1995).

Essential Nutrients

An individual needs to ingest more than 40 different nutrients to maintain good health. Because no single food source contains all of these nutrients, variety in one's diet is essential. Eating a wide variety of foods will help ensure adequate intake of carbohydrates, fats, proteins, vitamins, and minerals.

Carbohydrates

Carbohydrates should be the body's main source of fuel. Between 55-60% of an individual's diet should be composed of carbohydrates. Of this 55-60%, 45-50% of total daily caloric intake should be from complex carbohydrates, leaving simple carbohydrates to account for less than 10% of that individual's daily carbohydrate intake.

Complex carbohydrates are relatively low in calories (4 cal./gr.), nutritionally dense, and are a rich source of vitamins, minerals, and water. Complex carbohydrates provide the body with a steady source of energy for hours. The best sources of complex carbohydrates are breads, cereals, pastas, and grains.

Dietary fiber, also known as roughage or bulk, is a type of complex carbohydrate that is present mainly in leaves, roots, skins and seeds. Dietary fiber is the part of the plant that is not digested in the small intestine, and it helps decrease the risk of cardiovascular disease, cancer, and may lower an individual's risk of coronary heart disease.

Dietary fiber is either soluble or insoluble. *Soluble fiber* dissolves in water. It helps the body excrete fats and has been shown to reduce levels of blood cholesterol and blood sugar, while also helping to control diabetes. Water soluble fiber travels through the digestive tract in gel-like form, pacing the absorption of cholesterol, which helps prevent dramatic shifts in blood sugar levels. Soluble fiber is found primarily in oats, fruits, barley, and legumes.

Insoluble fiber does not dissolve easily in water; therefore, it cannot be digested by the body. Insoluble fiber causes softer, bulkier stool that increases peristalsis. This, in turn, reduces the risk of colon cancer by allowing food residues to pass through the intestinal tract more quickly, limiting the exposure and absorption time of toxic substances within the waste materials. Primary sources of insoluble fiber include wheat, cereals, vegetables, and the skins of fruits.

TABLE 8.2. Good Sources of Dietary Fiber

Fruits	Grams
1 medium apple	4–5
1 banana	3
1 cup blueberries	5
10 dates	7
1 orange	3
1 pear	5
1 cup strawberries	3
1 watermelon slice	2–3

Vegetables	Grams
1 artichoke	4
1 raw carrot	2
1/2 cup cream style corn	6
1 cup chopped lettuce	1
1/2 cup green peas	6
1 cup cooked spinach	6
1 cup cooked squash	5–6
1 tomato	2

Legumes	Grams
1 cup cooked black beans	15
1 cup cooked green beans	3
1 cup pork and beans	8
1 cup cooked blackeyed peas	11
1 cup kidney beans	20
1 cup cooked navy beans	16
1 cup cooked pinto beans	9

Grains	Grams
1 bagel	1
1 whole grain slice of bread	1–
4 graham crackers	3
1 bran muffin	2
hot dog/hamburger bun	1
1 cup cooked oatmeal	7–9
1/2 cup Grape Nuts cereal	3.5
1 cup Nature Valley granola	7.5
3/4 cup Shredded Wheat cereal	4
1 cup cooked macaroni	1
1 cup cooked rice	2.5–4
1 cup cooked spaghetti	1–2

Other	Grams
1 cup almonds	15
1 cup cashews	8
1 cup shredded coconut	11
1 tbsp peanut butter	1
1/4 cup sunflower seeds	2

The recommended daily intake of fiber is 25-30 grams per day. Health disorders associated with low fiber intake include constipation, diverticulitis, hemorrhoids, gall bladder disease, and obesity. Problems associated with ingesting too much fiber include a loss of calcium, phosphorous, iron, and disturbances of the gastrointestinal system.

Simple carbohydrates are sugars that have little nutritive value beyond their energy content. Sugars that are found naturally in milk, fruit, honey, and some vegetables, are examples of simple carbohydrates. Foods high in simple sugars are sometimes dismissed as "empty calories," and examples of these foods include candy, cakes, jellies, and sodas.

Fats

Fats, which supply the body with 9 calories of energy per gram ingested, are the body's primary source of energy. While many Americans consume too many of their daily calories from fats (37-40%), dietary fat is not necessarily a "bad" component of an individual's diet at moderate levels of consumption. At moderate amounts, between 25-30% of daily calories, fat is crucial to good nutrition.

Fat has many essential functions, including: providing the body with stored energy, insulating the body to preserve body heat, contributing to cellular structure, and protecting vital organs by absorbing shock. Fat not only adds flavor and texture to foods and helps satisfy an individual's appetite because it is digested more slowly, it also supplies the body with essential fatty acids, and transports fat soluble vitamins A, E, D, and K. Fat is also necessary for normal growth and healthy skin, and is essential in the synthesis of certain hormones.

There are different types of dietary fat. *Saturated fats* are found primarily in animal products such as meats, lard, cream, butter, cheese, and whole milk. However, coconut and palm oils are two plant sources of saturated fat. A defining characteristic of saturated fats is that they typically do not melt at room temperature (an exception being the above mentioned oils that are "almost solid" at room temperature). Saturated fats do increase an individual's blood cholesterol level and are a contributor to colorectal cancer.

Unsaturated fats are derived primarily from plant products. *Monounsaturated fats* are found in foods such as olives, peanuts, and canola oil, peanut oil, and olive oil. *Polyunsaturated fats* are found in margarine, pecans, corn oil, cottonseed oil, sunflower oil, and soybean oil.

Fats become counterproductive to good health when they are consumed in excess. Too much fat in many American's diets are the reason Americans lead the world in heart disease. Excess fat intake elevates blood cholesterol levels and leads to atherosclerosis, or a hardening of the arteries. 30-40% of all cancers in men, and 60% of all cancers in women, have been attributed to diets with excess fat, and have also been linked to cancer of the breast, colon, and prostate more frequently than any other dietary factor.

Protein

While proteins should make up only 12-15% of total calories ingested, they are the essential "building blocks" of the body. They are needed for the growth, maintenance, and repair of all body tissues, i.e. muscles, blood, bones, internal organs, skin, hair, and nails. Proteins also help maintain the normal balance of body fluids and are needed to make enzymes, hormones, and antibodies that fight infection.

Proteins are made up of approximately twenty amino acids. An individual's body uses all twenty of these amino acids in the formation of different proteins. Eleven of the twenty are *non-essential amino acids*—they are manufactured in the body if food proteins in a person's diet provide enough nitrogen. Nine of the twenty are *essential amino acids*—the body cannot produce these, and thus must be supplied through an individual's diet. All amino acids must be present at the same time for particular protein synthesis to occur.

45-65 grams per day is the suggested RDA of protein for adults (intake should not exceed 1.6 gr./kg. of body weight (kg. = 2.2 lbs.)). A few exceptions to this rule should be noted: overweight individuals need slightly less than the calculated "norm," and women who are pregnant or lactating need slightly more protein per pound of body weight than the calculation indicates.

It is inadvisable to consume more protein than the daily recommended dosage (45-65 gr./day), particularly in the form of protein supplements. Excessive protein supplementation can damage the kidneys, increase calcium excretion, negatively affect bone health, and inhibit muscle growth and endurance performance.

TABLE 8.3. Percentage of Fat Calories in Foods

Type of food	Less Than 15% of Calories from Fat	15%–30% of Calories from Fat	30%–50% of Calories from Fat	More Than 50% of Calories from Fat
Fruits and Vegetables	Fruits, plain vegetables, juices, pickles, sauerkraut		French fries, hash browns	Avocados, coconuts, olives
Bread and Cereals	Grains and flours, most breads, most cereals, corn tortillas, pitas, matzoh, bagels, noodles and pasta	Corn bread, flour tortillas, oatmeal, soft rolls and buns, wheat germ	Breakfast bars, biscuits and muffins, granola, pancakes and waffles, donuts, taco shells, pastries, croissants	
Dairy Products	Nonfat milk, dry curd cottage cheese, nonfat cottage cheese, nonfat yogurt	Buttermilk, low-fat yogurt, 1% milk, low-fat cottage cheese	Whole milk, 2% milk, creamed cottage cheese	Butter, cream, sour cream, half & half, most cheeses, (including part-skim and lite cheeses)
Meats		Beef round; veal loin, round, and shoulder; pork tenderloin	Beef and veal, lamb, fresh and picnic hams	All ground beef, spareribs, cold cuts, beef, hot dogs, pastrami
Poultry	Egg whites	Chicken and turkey (light meat without skin)	Chicken and turkey (light meat with skin, dark meat without skin), duck and goose (without skin)	Chicken/turkey (dark meat with skin), chicken/turkey hot dogs and bologna, egg yolks, whole eggs
Seafood	Clams, cod, crab, crawfish, flounder, haddock, lobster, perch, sole, scallops, shrimp, tuna (in water)	Bass and sea bass, halibut, mussels, oyster, tuna (fresh)	Anchovies, catfish, salmon, sturgeon, trout, tuna (in oil, drained)	Herring, mackerel, sardines
Beans and Nuts	Dried beans and peas, chestnuts, water chestnuts		Soybeans	Tofu, most nuts and seeds, peanut butter
Fats and Oils	Oil-free and some lite salad dressings			Butter, margarine, all mayonnaise (including reduced-calorie), most salad dressings, all oils
Soups	Bouillons, broths consomme	Most soups	Cream soups, bean soups, "just add water" noodle soups	Cheddar cheese soups, New England clam chowder
Desserts	Angel food cake, gelatin, some new fat-free cakes	Pudding, tapioca	Most cakes, most pies	
Frozen Desserts	Sherbert, low-fat frozen yogurt, sorbet, fruit ices	Ice milk	Frozen yogurt	All ice cream
Snack foods	Popcorn (air popped), pretzels, rye crackers, rice cakes, fig bars, raisin biscuit cookies, marshmallows, most hard candy, fruit rolls	Lite microwave popcorn, Scandinavian "crisps," plain crackers, caramels, fudge, gingersnaps, graham crackers	Snack crackers, popcorn (popped in oil), cookies, candy bars, granola bars	Most microwave popcorn, corn and potato chips, chocolate, buttery crackers

SOURCE: American Heart Association/USDA.

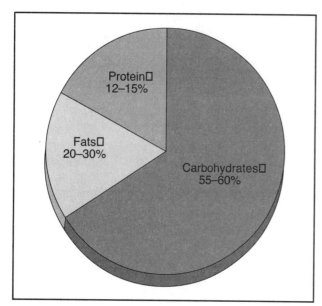

Protein
12–15%

Fats
20–30%

Carbohydrates
55–60%

From *A Wellness Way of Life*, Fourth Edition by Robbins et al. Copyright © 1999. Reproduced with permission of The McGraw-Hill Companies.

Figure 8.1 Daily Diet Recommendations

Vitamins

Vitamins are necessary for normal body metabolism, growth, and development. They do not provide the body with energy, but they do allow the energy from consumed carbohydrates, fats, and proteins to be released. Although vitamins are vital to life, they are required in minute amounts. Due primarily to adequate food supply, vitamin deficiencies in Americans are rare. However, there are some situations that may alter an individual's requirements, including pregnancy and smoking. Non-smokers need to consume 60 mg of Vitamin C each day; to get the same nutritional benefits, a smoker must ingest 100 mg of Vitamin C each day. A man or a non-pregnant woman should consume 180-200 mg. of folic acid, while a pregnant woman should consume approximately 400mg. of folic acid per day.

Vitamins are grouped as either fat-soluble or water-soluble. *Fat-soluble vitamins* are transported by the body's fat cells and by the liver. They include vitamins A, E, D, and K. Fat-soluble vitamins are not excreted in urine; therefore, they are stored in the body for relatively long periods of time (many months), and can build up to potentially toxic levels if excessive doses are consumed over time.

Water-soluble vitamins include the B vitamins and vitamin C. These vitamins are not stored in the body for a significant amount of time, and amounts that are consumed and not used relatively quickly by the body are excreted through urine and sweat. For this reason, water-soluble vitamins must be replaced daily. Table 8.4 summarizes the functions of vitamins, lists the best sources for each vitamin, and outlines associated deficiency symptoms.

Minerals

Minerals are inorganic substances that are critical to many enzyme functions in the body. Approximately 25 minerals have important roles in bodily functions. Minerals are contained in all cells and are concentrated in hard parts of the body—nails, teeth, and bones. They are crucial to maintaining water balance and the acid-base balance. Minerals are essential components of respiratory pigments, enzymes and enzyme systems, while also regulating muscular and nervous tissue excitability, blood clotting, and normal heart rhythm. Table 8.5 outlines the major sources and functions of specific minerals, as well as listing deficiency symptoms for those minerals.

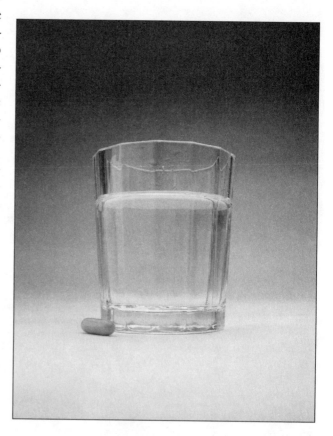

TABLE 8.4. Facts About Vitamins

Vitamin	Major Functions	Signs of Prolonged Deficiency	Toxic Effects of Megadoses	Important Dietary Sources
Fat-Soluble Vitamin A	Maintenance of eyes, vision, skin, linings of the nose, mouth, digestive and urinary tracts, immune function	Night blindness; dry, scaling skin; increased susceptibility to infection; loss of appetite; anemia; kidney stones	Headache, vomiting and diarrhea, dryness of mucous membranes, vertigo, double vision, bone abnormalities, liver damage, miscarriage and birth defects, convulsions, coma, respiratory failure	Liver, milk, butter, cheese, and fortified margarine; carrots, spinach, cantaloupe, and other orange and deep-green vegetables and fruits contain carotenes that the body converts to vitamin A
Vitamin D	Aid in calcium and phosphorus metabolism, promote calcium absorption, develop & maintain bones and teeth	Rickets (bone deformities) in children; bone softening, loss, and fractures in adults	Calcium deposits in kidneys and blood vessels, causing irreversible kidney and cardiovascular damage	Fortified milk & margarine, fish liver oils, butter, egg yolks (sunlight on skin also produces vitamin D)
Vitamin E	Protection and maintenance of cellular membranes	Red blood cell breakage and anemia, weakness, neurological problems, muscle cramps	Relatively nontoxic, but may cause excess bleeding or formation of blood clots	Vegetable oils, whole grains, nuts and seeds, green leafy vegetables, asparagus, peaches; smaller amounts widespread in other foods
Vitamin K	Production of factors essential for blood clotting	Hemorrhaging	None observed	Green leafy vegetables; smaller amounts widespread in other foods
Water-Soluble Vitamin C	Maintenance and repair of connective tissue, bones, teeth, and cartilage; promotion of healing; aid in iron absorption	Scurvy (weakening of collagenous structures resulting in widespread capillary hemorrhaging), anemia, reduced resistance to infection, bleeding gums, weakness, loosened teeth, rough skin, joint pain, poor wound healing, hair loss, poor iron absorption	Urinary stones in some people, acid stomach from ingesting supplements in pill form, nausea, diarrhea, headache, fatigue	Peppers, broccoli, spinach, brussels sprouts, citrus fruits, strawberries, tomatoes, potatoes, cabbage, other fruits and vegetables
Thiamin	Conversion of carbohydrates into usable forms of energy, maintenance of appetite and nervous system function	Beriberi (symptoms include edema or muscle wasting, mental confusion, anorexia, enlarged heart, abnormal heart rhythm, muscle degeneration and weakness, nerve changes)	None reported	Yeast, whole-grain and enriched breads and cereals, organ meats, liver, pork, lean meats, poultry, eggs, fish, beans, nuts, legumes
Riboflavin	Energy metabolism; maintenance of skin, mucous membranes, and nervous system structures	Cracks at corners of mouth, sore throat, skin rash, hypersensitivity to light, purple tongue	None reported	Dairy products, whole-grain and enriched breads and cereals, lean meats, poultry, green vegetables, liver
Niacin	Converting carbohydrates fats, and protein into usable forms of energy; essential for growth, hormone synthesis	Pellagra (symptoms include weakness, diarrhea, dermatitis, inflammation of mucous membranes, mental illness)	Flushing of the skin, nausea, vomiting, diarrhea, changes in the metabolism of glycogen and fatty acids	Eggs, chicken, turkey, fish, milk, whole grains, nuts, enriched breads and cereals, lean meats, legumes*
Vitamin B-6	Enzyme reactions involving amino acids and the metabolism of carbohydrates, lipids, and nucleic acids	Anemia, convulsions, cracks at corners of mouth, dermatitis, nausea, confusion	Neurological abnormalities and damage	Eggs, poultry, whole grains, nuts, legumes, liver, kidney, pork
Folate	Amino acid metabolism, synthesis of RNA and DNA, new cell synthesis	Anemia, gastrointestinal disturbances, decreased resistance to infection, depression	Diarrhea, reduction of zinc absorption, possible kidney enlargement and damage	Green leafy vegetables, yeast, oranges, whole grains, legumes, liver
Vitamin B-12	Synthesis of red & white blood cells; other metabolic reactions	Anemia, fatigue, nervous system damage, sore tongue	None reported	Eggs, milk, meat, liver
Biotin	Metabolism of fats, carbohydrates, and proteins	Rash, nausea, vomiting, weight loss depression, fatigue, hair loss; not known under natural circumstances	None reported	Cereals, yeast, nuts, cheese, egg yolks, soy flour, liver; widespread foods
Pantothenic acid	Metabolism of fats, carbohydrates, and proteins	Fatigue, numbness & tingling of hands and feet, gastrointestinal disturbance; not known under natural circumstances	Diarrhea, water retention	Peanuts, whole grains, legumes, fish, eggs, liver, kidney; smaller amounts found in milk, vegetables, and fruits

*Niacin can be made in the body from trytophan, so this list includes foods containing niacin and/or tryptophan.

From *Fitness for Living* by Hyman et al. Copyright © 1999 by Kendall/Hunt Publishing Company. Reprinted by permission.

TABLE 8.5. Facts About Selected Minerals

Mineral	Major Functions	Signs of Prolonged Deficiency	Toxic Effects of Megadoses	Important Dietary Sources
Calcium	Maintenance of bones and teeth, blood clotting, maintenance of cell membranes, control of nerve impulses and muscle contraction	Stunted growth in children, bone mineral loss in adults	Nausea, vomiting, hypertension, constipation, urinary stones, calcium deposits in soft tissues, inhibition of absorption of certain minerals	Milk and milk products, tofu, fortified orange juice and bread, green leafy vegetables, bones in fish
Fluoride	Maintenance of tooth (and possibly bone) structure	Higher frequency of tooth decay	Increased bone density, mottling of teeth, impaired kidney function, neurological disturbances	Fluoride-containing drinking water, tea, marine fish eaten with bones
Iron	Component of hemoglobin (carries oxygen to tissues), myoglobin (in muscle fibers), and enzymes	Iron-deficiency anemia, weakness, impaired immune function, cold hands and feet, gastrointestinal distress	Iron deposits in soft tissues, causing liver and kidney damage, joint pains, sterility, and disruption of cardiac function	Lean meats, legumes, enriched flour, green vegetables, dried fruit, liver; absorption is enhanced by presence of vitamin C
Iodine	Essential part of thyroid hormones, regulation of body metabolism	Goiter (enlarged thyroid), cretinism (birth defect)	Depression of thyroid activity, hyperthyroidism in susceptible individuals	Iodized salt, seafood
Magnesium	Transmission of nerve impulses, bone and tooth structure, energy transfer composition of many enzyme systems	Neurological disturbances, impaired immune function, kidney disorders, nausea, weight loss, growth failure in children	Nausea, vomiting, central nervous system depression, coma; death in people with impaired kidney function	Widespread in foods and water (except soft water); especially found in wheat bran, milk products, legumes, nuts, seeds, leafy vegetables
Phosphorus	Bone growth and maintenance (combined with calcium), energy transfer in cells	Weakness, bone loss, kidney disorders, cardiorespiratory failure	Drop in blood calcium levels	Present in nearly all foods, especially milk, cheese, cereal, legumes, meats
Potassium	Nerve function and body water balance	Muscular weakness, nausea, drowsiness, paralysis, confusion, disruption of cardiac rhythm	Cardiac arrest	Meats, milk, fruits, vegetables, grains, legumes
Sodium	Body water balance, acid-base balance, nerve function	Muscle weakness, loss of appetite, nausea, vomiting; sodium deficiency is rarely seen	Edema, hypertension in sensitive people	Salt, soy sauce, salted foods
Zinc	Enzyme reactions, including synthesis of proteins, RNA, and DNA; wound healing; immune response; ability to taste	Growth failure, reproductive failure, loss of appetite, impaired taste acuity, skin rash, impaired immune function, poor wound healing, night blindness	Vomiting, impaired immune function, decline in serum HDL levels, impaired magnesium absorption	Whole grains, meat, eggs, liver, seafood (especially oysters)

From *Fitness for Living* by Hyman et al. Copyright © 1999 by Kendall/Hunt Publishing Company. Reprinted by permission.

Two groups of minerals are necessary in an individual's diet: macrominerals and microminerals. *Macrominerals* are the seven minerals the body needs in relatively large quantities (100 mg. or more each day.) In most cases, these minerals can be acquired by eating a variety of foods each day, and they include calcium, chloride, magnesium, phosphorus, potassium, sodium, and sulfur.

While *Microminerals* are essential to healthy living, they are needed in smaller quantities (less than 100 mg. per day) than macrominerals. Examples of these minerals include chromium, cobalt, copper, fluoride, iodine, iron, manganese, molybdenum, selenium, and zinc.

Antioxidants

Antioxidants are compounds that come to the aid of every cell in the body facing an ongoing barrage of damage resulting from daily oxygen exposure, environmental pollution, chemicals and pesticides,

TABLE 8.6.	Antioxidants and Their Primary Food Sources
Vitamin A	Fortified milk; egg yolk; cheese; liver; butter; fish oil; dark green, yellow, and orange vegetables and fruits
Vitamin C	Papaya, cantaloupe, melons, citrus fruits, grapefruit, strawberries, raspberries, kiwi, cauliflower, tomatoes, dark green vegetables, green and red peppers, asparagus, broccoli, cabbage, collard greens, orange juice and tomato juice
Vitamin E	Vegetable oils, nuts and seeds, dried beans, egg yolk, green leafy vegetables, sweet potatoes, wheat germ, 100% whole wheat bread, 100% whole grain cereal, oatmeal, mayonnaise
Carotenoids	Sweet potatoes, carrots, squash, tomatoes, asparagus, broccoli, spinach, romaine lettuce, mango, cantaloupe, pumpkin, apricots, peaches, papaya
Flavenoids	Purple grapes, wine, apples, berries, peas, beets, onions, garlic, green tea
Selenium	Lean meat, seafood, kidney, liver, dairy products, 100% whole grain cereal, 100% whole wheat bread

additives in processed foods, stress hormones, and sun radiation. Studies continue to show the ability of antioxidants to suppress cell deterioration and "slow" the aging process. Realizing the potential power of these substances should encourage Americans to take action by eating at least five servings of a wide variety of fruits and vegetables each day.

There are many proven health benefits of antioxidants. Vitamin C speeds the healing process, helps prevent infection, and prevents scurvy. Vitamin E helps prevent heart disease by stopping the oxidation of low-density lipoprotein (the harmful form of cholesterol), strengthens the immune system, and may play a role in the prevention of Alzheimer's disease, cataracts, and some forms of cancer, providing further proof of the benefits of antioxidants.

Water

In many cases, water is the "forgotten nutrient." Although water does not provide energy to the body in the form of calories, it is a substance that is essential to life. Among other things, water lubricates joints, absorbs shock, regulates body temperature, maintains blood volume, and transports fluids throughout the body, while comprising 60% of an individual's body.

While it is clear that adequate hydration is crucial to proper physiological functioning, many people are in a semi-hydrated state most of the time.

Whether exercising or not, hydration should be a continuous process. Prolonged periods of dehydration can result in as much as a ten percent loss of intracellular water concentration, and can result in death. Individuals more susceptible to dehydration include: persons who are overweight, deconditioned, or unacclimitized to heat, the very old and the very young, and individuals who do not eat breakfast or drink water.

To ensure proper water balance and prevent dehydration, approximately six to eight eight-ounce glasses of water should be consumed each day an individual is not exercising. When working out, current recommendations for water intake are 2 to 3 eight-ounce cups of water before exercising, 4–6 oz. of cool water every 15 minutes during the workout, and rehydrating after the activity.

The Food Guide Pyramid

Created in 1992 by the Federal Government, the Food Guide Pyramid is an attempt to arm more Americans with the knowledge that will allow them to create a healthy, balanced, and tasty diet. A visual representation of the Food Guide Pyramid is seen in figure 8.2.

The Bread Group

Foods from the bread group are a great source of energy, providing the body with complex carbohydrates. Starchy foods, such as these, are not fatten-

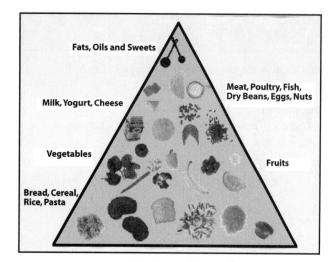

Figure 8.2 The Food Guide Pyramid

ing if butter, cheese, or other creamy sauces are not added to them. Selections of whole grain products from this group will also help an individual to maximize the intake of fiber and other nutrients.

Examples of foods within this group include: bread, cereal, pasta, and rice. 6–11 servings are the suggested number of daily servings from the bread group. Examples of serving equivalents within this group are as follows: 1 serving = 1 slice of bread, 1oz. of ready to eat cereal, or ½ cup of cooked cereal, rice, or pasta.

The Fruit Group

Fruits are a rich source of vitamins, the most notable of which is Vitamin C. Most fruits are naturally low in fat and calories. By selecting fresh fruits and fruit juices, and frozen, canned, or dried fruits, and avoiding fruits processed with sugar-sweetened juices and syrups, an individual can significantly decrease unwanted or unintended fat and calories in their diet.

Apples, oranges, bananas, melons, and berries are excellent examples of foods contained within the fruit group. Current recommendations for the number of servings each day from this group are 2–3. Serving equivalents for the fruit group are: 1 serving = 1 medium apple, banana, or orange, 1 melon wedge, ½ cup of chopped fruits or berries, or ¾ cup of fruit juice.

The Vegetable Group

Vegetables are an excellent source of natural fiber, low in fat, and provide the body with vitamins,

especially Vitamins A and C. For maximum nutritional benefits, an individual should consume dark leafy green vegetables, deep orange or yellow vegetables, or starchy vegetables such as potatoes or yams.

Examples of foods within this group include: carrots, peas, potatoes, yams, squash, green beans, broccoli, cauliflower, and corn. 3–5 servings from this group each day is recommended. 1 serving from the vegetable group = 1 cup of raw, leafy, greens, ½ cup of other chopped vegetables, or ¾ cup of vegetable juice.

The Meat Group

Animal sources of foods, as well as beans, nuts, and seeds are all found within the meat group and are excellent sources of protein, iron, zinc, and B Vitamins. It is important for individuals to be aware when making their food selections that some of the foods found within this group can be relatively high in fat content, especially saturated fats. Lower fat alternatives within this group include fish, poultry, lean cuts of beef, beans, and peas.

Red meats, poultry, pork, fish, dry beans, eggs, and nuts are all examples of food found within the meat group. Two to three servings are the suggested number of daily servings from the meat group. Serving equivalents for the meat group are as follows: 1 serving = 2–3 oz. of cooked lean meat, poultry, or fish, 1 egg, ½ cup of cooked beans, or 2 tablespoons of seeds or nuts.

The Milk Group

Milk products are the best source of calcium. These products also provide protein and Vitamin B-12. Because these foods can be high in fat and calories, it is best to choose low fat varieties of these foods to keep calories, cholesterol, and saturated fat to a minimum.

Examples of foods found within the milk group include: milk, yogurt, and cheese. Current recommendations for the number of servings each day from this group are 2–3. 1 serving from the milk group = 1 cup of milk or yogurt, or 1½ oz. of cheese.

The Fat Group

Foods found within this group are typically high in fat, sugars, and "empty" calories. These foods generally taste great and do provide the body with calories. However, they do very little else nutritionally. Exceptions to this rule include vegetable oil, which is a rich source of Vitamin E and molasses, an excellent source of iron.

Cookies, candies, sodas, and oils are examples of foods found within this group. The suggested daily servings for this group are that they should be used sparingly and in moderation. There are no set serving equivalents for this food group.

Other Issues in Nutrition

Reading Labels

Beginning in May of 1993, the federal government has required food manufacturers to provide accurate nutritional information about their products on their product labels. Because these food labels are standardized, relatively straight forward and easy to read, much of the guess work has been taken out of good nutrition.

Ingredients are listed on food labels by percentage of total weight, in order from highest to lowest. By simply reading the listing of ingredients, an individual can determine if a food is relatively high in fat, sugar, salt, etc.

Food labels are required, by law, to include the number of servings per container and number of calories per serving. They must also list the amount per serving and the percentage of the daily value of total fat (including saturated fat), cholesterol, sodium, total carbohydrates (including dietary fiber and sugars), protein, vitamins, and minerals. Figure 8.3 provides an example of the required nutrition information found on packaged foods.

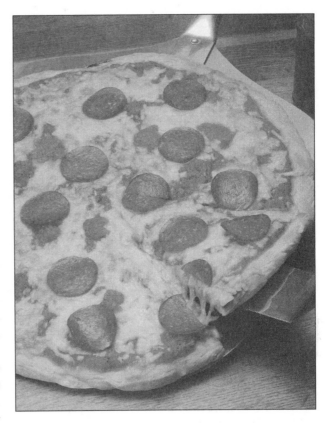

Fast Foods / Eating Out

Today, people eat meals outside of their homes more often than ever before. Due to their quick service and comparatively low prices, fast food chains are the most frequent source for meals prepared outside of the home. Each day, millions of people line up inside or drive through outside service lanes of 1 of the over 140,000 fast food establishments in this country.

When meals are prepared with speed and convenience as the primary focus, good nutrition will, in most cases, suffer. A great majority of fast foods are high in fat, calories, and salt, and low in many of the essential nutrients and dietary fiber.

However, fast food does not have to mean "junk food." While it may take a little more thought and discretion, quick and healthy alternatives do exist. Depending on what ingredients are used and how the food is prepared, fast foods served in restaurants can be healthy. Many restaurants have nutritional information about the foods they serve posted within the dining area or on their menus. By taking a couple of extra minutes to think about their best and most nutritious options, an individual can make dining out more nutritious, filling, and healthy.

Dietary Supplements

The best and most preferred method of ingesting an adequate supply of the proper nutrients is to eat a healthy diet consisting of at least five servings of fruits and vegetables. Dietary supplements provide a means to deliver these nutrients to your body in a more convenient, but often less effective, form. For individuals that are considering a dietary supplement, it would be prudent to consult a knowledgeable health professional prior to beginning supplementation. Taken in concentrations higher than the recommended daily allowance, some nutrients have undesirable side effects—some are even toxic.

Many individuals considering dietary supplementation are of the mind set "if one (or one hun-

Serving Size

Is your serving the same size as the one on the label? If you eat double the serving size listed, you need to double the nutrient and calorie values. If you eat one-half the serving size shown here, cut the nutrient and calorie values in half.

Calories

Are you overweight? Cut back a little on calories! Look here to see how a serving of the food adds to your daily total. A 5'4", 138-lb. active woman needs about 2,200 calories each day. A 5'10", 174-lb. active man needs about 2,900. How about you?

Total Carbohydrate

When you cut down on fat, you can eat more carbohydrates. Carbohydrates are in foods like bread, potatoes, fruits and vegetables. Choose these often! They give you more nutrients than **sugars** like soda pop and candy.

Dietary Fiber

Grandmother called it "roughage," but her advice to eat more is still up-to-date! That goes for both soluble and in-soluble kinds of dietary fiber. Fruits, vegetables, whole-grain foods, beans and peas are all good sources and can help reduce the risk of heart disease and cancer.

Protein

Most Americans get more protein than they need. Where there is animal protein, there is also fat and cholesterol. Eat small servings of lean meat, fish and poultry. Use skim or low-fat milk, yogurt and cheese. Try vegetable proteins like beans, grains and cereals.

Vitamins & Minerals

Your goal here is 100% of each for the day. Don't count on one food to do it all. Let a combination of foods add up to a winning score.

Nutrition Facts

Serving Size $1/2$ cup (114g)
Servings Per Container 4

Amount Per Serving

Calories 90   Calories from Fat 30

	% Daily Value*
Total Fat 3g	**5%**
Saturated Fat 0g	**0%**
Cholesterol 0mg	**0%**
Sodium 300mg	**13%**
Total Carbohydrate 13g	**4%**
Dietary Fiber 3g	**12%**
Sugars 3g	
Protein 3g	

Vitamin A	80%	•	Vitamin C	60%
Calcium	4%	•	Iron	4%

*Percent Daily Values are based on a 2000 calorie diet. Your daily values may be higher or lower depending on your calorie needs:

	Calories	2000	2500
Total Fat	Less than	65g	80g
Sat Fat	Less than	20g	25g
Cholesterol	Less than	300mg	300mg
Sodium	Less than	2400mg	2400mg
Total Carbohydrate		300g	375g
Fiber		25g	30g

Calories per gram:
Fat 9 • Carbohydrates 4 • Protein 4

More nutrients may be listed on some labels.

Total Fat

Aim low. Most people need to cut back on fat! Too much fat may contribute to heart disease and cancer. Try to limit your **calories from fat**. For a healthy heart, choose foods with a big difference between the total number of calories and the number of calories from fat.

Saturated Fat

A new kind of fat? No—saturated fat is part of the total fat in food. It is listed separately because it's the key player in raising blood cholesterol and your risk of heart disease. Eat less!

Cholesterol

Too much cholesterol—a second cousin to fat— can lead to heart disease. Challenge yourself to eat less than 300 mg each day.

Sodium

You call it "salt," the label calls it "sodium." Either way, it may add up to high blood pressure in some people. So, keep your sodium intake low—2,400 to 3,000 mg or less each day.*

*The AHA recommends no more than 3,000 mg sodium per day for healthy adults.

Daily Value

Feel like you're drowning in numbers? Let the Daily Value be your guide. Daily Values are listed for people who eat 2,000 or 2,500 calories each day. If you eat more, your personal daily value may be higher than what's listed on the label. If you eat less, your personal daily value may be lower.

For fat, saturated fat, cholesterol and sodium, choose foods with a low % **Daily Value**. For total carbohydrate, dietary fiber, vitamins and minerals, your daily value goal is to reach 100% of each.

g = grams (About 28 g = 1 ounce)
mg = milligrams (1,000 mg = 1 g)

You Can Rely on the New Label

Rest assured, when you see key words and health claims on product labels, they mean what they say as defined by the government. For example:

Key Words	What They Mean
Fat Free	Less than 0.5 gram of fat per serving
Low Fat	3 grams of fat (or less) per serving
Lean	Less than 10 grams of fat, 4 grams of saturated fat and 95 milligrams of cholesterol per serving
Light (Lite)	$1/3$ less calories or no more than $1/2$ the fat of the higher-calorie, higher-fat version; or no more than $1/2$ the sodium of the higher-sodium version
Cholesterol Free	Less than 2 milligrams of cholesterol and 2 grams (or less) of saturated fat per serving

To Make	The Food
Health Claims About… Heart Disease and Fats	Must Be … Low in fat, saturated fat and cholesterol
Blood Pressure and Sodium	Low in sodium
Heart Disease and Fruits, Vegetables and Grain Products	A fruit, vegetable or grain product low in fat, saturated fat and cholesterol, that contains at least 0.6 gram soluble fiber, without fortification, per serving

Other claims may appear on some labels.

Figure 8.3 Food Label: Nutrition Facts

dred, etc.) is good, then two will be twice as good!" There is no scientific evidence that this is true. To the contrary, in many cases, excesses of certain nutrients, especially fat-soluble vitamins A, E, D, and K, can become detrimental to the body and can potentially reach toxic levels. Kidney and liver damage, among other health problems, can occur from megadoses of these fat-soluble vitamins and certain minerals. Megadosing on certain vitamins or minerals can also interfere with the absorption of other vital nutrients. For these reasons, consuming more than the recommended daily allowance of vitamins and minerals is discouraged.

There are specific instances in an individual's life when dietary supplementation might be advisable (i.e. pregnancy, anemia and other medical conditions, or certain types of vegetarianism.) However, it is recommended that consultation with a registered dietitian or physician occur prior to beginning supplementation, regardless of the situation.

Vegetarianism

There have always been people who, for one reason or another (religious, ethical, or philosophical), have chosen to follow a vegetarian diet. However, in recent years, a vegetarian diet has become increasingly popular.

There are four different types of vegetarian diets. *Vegans* are considered true vegetarians. Their diets contain absolutely no meat, chicken, fish, eggs, or milk products. Their primary sources of protein are vegetables, fruits, and grains. Because Vitamin B12 is normally found only in meat products, many vegans choose to supplement their diet with this vitamin.

Lactovegetarians eat dairy products, fruits, and vegetables but do not consume any other animal products (meat, poultry, fish, or eggs.)

Ovolactovegetarians are another type of vegetarians. They eat eggs as well as dairy products, fruits, and vegetables, but still do not consume meat, poultry, and or fish.

A person who eats fruits, vegetables, dairy products, eggs, and a small selection of poultry, fish, and other seafood is a partial or *semivegetarian*. These individuals do not consume any beef or pork.

Vegetarians of all four types can meet all their nutritional needs through their daily food intake. Because they have chosen to omit certain nutritional sources, it is critical that they eat a wide variety of the foods from their available sources and limit their consumption of sweets and fatty foods. With deliberate and mindful food selections and consumption, a vegetarian diet can be a healthy low-fat alternative to a more typical American diet.

Body Composition

Body composition is one of the five components of health-related fitness (see chapter 2 for the other four components: cardiovascular endurance, muscular endurance, muscular strength, and flexibility).

An individual's *body composition* measures their percentage of body fat in relation to their percentage of lean body mass (muscle, bone and internal organs). This ratio of body fat to lean body mass is a much better indicator of overall fitness or health than a person's actual body weight.

Current thinking suggests an ideal standard of 18–23 percent body fat for women and 7–15 percent body fat for men. By maintaining a health body composition, individuals protect themselves against chronic diseases such as heart disease, stroke, and adult-onset diabetes.

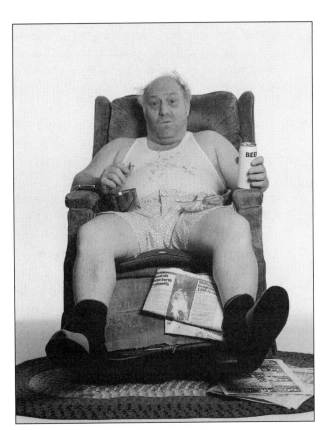

Guidelines for a Successful Weight Loss Program

The American College of Sports Medicine has put together the following eleven guidelines in an effort to help individuals recognize potentially successful weight loss programs and avoid unsound or dangerous weight loss programs.

1. Prolonged fasting and diet programs that severely restrict caloric intake are scientifically unsound and can be medically dangerous.

2. Fasting and diet programs that severely restrict caloric intake result in the loss of large amounts of water, electrolytes, minerals, glycogen stores, and other fat-free tissues, but with minimal amounts of fat loss.

3. Mild caloric restriction (500–1000 calories less than usual per day) results in smaller loss of water, electrolytes, minerals, and other fat-free tissues and is less likely to result in malnutrition.

4. Dynamic exercise of large muscle groups helps to maintain fat-free tissue, including lean muscle mass and bone density, and can result in a loss of body weight (primarily body fat).

5. A nutritionally sound diet resulting in mild caloric intake restrictions, coupled with an endurance exercise program, along with behavior modification of existing eating habits, is recommended for weight reduction. The rate of weight loss should never exceed 2 lbs. per week.

6. To maintain proper weight control and optimal body fat levels, a lifetime commitment to proper eating habits and regular physical activity is required.

7. A successful weight loss plan can be followed anywhere—at home, work, restaurants, parties, etc.

8. For a plan to be successful, the emphasis must be on portion size.

9. Successful weight loss plans incorporate a wide variety of nutritious foods that are easily accessible in the supermarket.

10. A weight loss plan must not be too costly if it is to be successful.

11. The most essential aspect of a weight loss program is that it can be followed for the rest of an individual's life.

Eating Disorders

Eating disorders are medically identifiable, potentially life threatening, mental health conditions related to obsessive eating patterns. Eating disorders are not new—descriptions of self-starvation have been found as far back as medieval times.

While more and more men are succumbing to eating disorders each year, this mental health con-

Ways to Love Your Body

- Become aware of what your body does each day, as the instrument of your life, not just an ornament for others.
- Think of your body as a tool. Create a list of all the things you can do with this body.
- Walk with your head held high, supported by pride and confidence in yourself as a person.
- Do something that will let you enjoy your body. Stretch, dance, walk, sing, take a bubble bath, get a massage.
- Wear comfortable styles that you really like and feel good in.
- Decide what you would rather do with the hours you waste every day criticizing your body.
- Describe 10 positive things about yourself without mentioning your appearance.
- Say to yourself "Life is too short to waste my time hating my body this way."
- Don't let your weight or shape keep you from doing things you enjoy.
- Create a list of people who have contributed to your life, your community, the world. Was their appearance important to their success and accomplishment? If not, why should yours be?
- If you had only one year to live, how important would your body image and appearance be?

By Margo Maine, Ph.D.
and
Eating Disorders' Awareness and Prevention

Courtesy of the Massachusetts Eating Disorder Association.

dition is typically thought of as a woman's disease. Unfortunately, even grade school girls can feel pressure to fit in or look thin. This can be very troubling and disruptive to young girls struggling to build a positive body image.

Typically, a person with an eating disorder seeks perfection and control over their life. Both anorexics and bulimics tend to suffer from low self-esteem and depression. They often have a conflict between a desire for perfection and feelings of personal inadequacy. This person typically has a distorted view of themselves, in that when they look into a mirror, they see themselves differently than others see them. Narcissism, or excessive vanity, is linked to both anorexia and bulimia.

Eating disorders are very serious and can be life threatening, with more people dying of anorexia than any other mental health disorder.

Types of Eating Disorders

Anorexia Nervosa is a state of starvation and emaciation usually resulting from severe dieting and excessive exercise. An anorexic will literally stop eating in an effort to control their size. Anorexic individuals can lose between 15–60% of their normal body weight, putting their body and their health in severe jeopardy.

Bulimia Nervosa is a process of bingeing and purging. This disorder is more common than anorexia nervosa. The purging is an attempt to control body weight, though bulimics seldom starve themselves as anorexics do. They have an intense fear of becoming overweight, and usually have episodes of secretive binge eating, followed by purging, frequent weight variations, and the inability to stop eating voluntarily. Bulimics often feel hunger, overeat, and then purge to rid themselves of the guilt of overeating.

Bulimia is often not fatal, but the medical health risks remain significant. Medical complications that can result from bulimia are esophageal inflammation, severe tooth decay, stomach rupture, reproductive problems and heart failure.

Fear of Obesity is an over-concern with thinness. It is less severe than anorexia, but can also have negative health consequences. This condition is often seen in achievement-oriented teenagers who seek to restrict their weight due to a fear of becoming obese. This condition can be a precursor to anorexia or bulimia if it is not detected and treated early.

Activity Nervosa is a condition where the individual suffers from the ever-present compulsion to exercise, regardless of illness or injury. The desire to exercise excessively may result in poor performance in other areas of that individual's life due to the resulting fatigue, weakness, and unhealthy body weight.

Who Is at Risk of Developing an Eating Disorder?

By far, more women than men succumb to eating disorders; however, the incidence of eating disorders in men is believed to be very underreported.

It is estimated that 1 in every 100 teenage girls is anorexic. Anorexia usually occurs in adolescent women (90% of all reported cases), although all age groups can be affected. It is estimated that one in every five college-bound females is bulimic.

Individuals living in economically developed nations, such as the United States, are much more likely to suffer from an eating disorder, due to the dual factors of an abundance of available food and external, societal pressure. College campuses have a higher incidence of people with eating disorders, while upper middle class women who are extremely self-critical are also more likely to become anorexic. Being aware of the groups at risk can be a large step towards prevention.

Activities such as dance and dance team, gymnastics, figure skating, track, and cheerleading, tend to have higher instances of eating disorders. An estimate of people suffering from anorexia and bulimia within these populations is 15–60%. Male wrestlers and body builders are also at risk due to the unsafe practice of attempting to shed pounds quickly in an attempt to "make weight" before a competition.

Causes of Eating Disorders

The causes of anorexia and bulimia are numerous and complex. Cultural factors, family pressure, psychological factors, emotional disorders, and chemical imbalances can all contribute to eating disorders.

Forty to eighty per cent of anorexics suffer from depression, as reduced levels of chemical neurotransmitters in the brain have been found in victims suffering from both eating disorders and depression. Links between hunger and depression have been discovered through research, which contributes to the depression a person with an eating disorder may feel.

For some bulimics, seasonality can adversely affect them, causing the disorder to worsen during the dark, winter months. Another startling statistic is that the onset of anorexia appears to peak in May, which is also the peak month for suicides.

Family factors are also critical. One study showed that 40% of all nine to ten year old girls were trying to lose weight, many at the encouragement of their mothers. Mothers of anorexics are often over-involved in their child's life, while bulimics' mothers are many times critical and detached.

It is clear that many people who suffer from eating disorders do not have a healthy body image. From an early age, there is enormous pressure in our culture from society, family, friends, the media, and often from one's self, to achieve the unachievable and unnecessary "perfect" body. A woman's self-worth is too often associated with other people's opinions, which in many cases put unrealistic emphasis on physical attractiveness.

Symptoms of Eating Disorders

Major weight loss is the most visible and the most common symptom of anorexia. Absent menstruation, dry skin, excessive hair on the skin, and thinning of scalp hair are also common in anorexic individuals. Gastrointestinal problems and orthopedic problems resulting from excessive exercise are also specific to this illness.

Bulimic individuals are often secretive and discreet, and are, therefore, often hard to identify. Typically, bulimics have a preoccupation with food, fluxuating between fantasies of food and guilt due to overeating. Symptoms of bulimia can include cuts and calluses on the finger joints from a person sticking their hands or fingers down their throat to induce vomiting, broken blood vessels around the eyes from the strain of vomiting, and damage to tooth enamel from stomach acid.

An extremely distorted body image is a very common symptom of both anorexia and bulimia.

Complications of Anorexia

The medical problems associated with anorexia are numerous and serious. Starvation damages bones, organs, muscles, the immune system, the digestive system, and the nervous system.

Between 5–20% of anorexics die due to suicide or other medical complications. Heart disease is the most common medical cause of death for people with severe anorexia.

Long term irregular or absent menstruation can cause sterility or bone loss. Severe anorexics also suffer nerve damage and may experience seizures. Anemia and gastrointestinal problems are also common to individuals suffering from this illness.

The most severe complication and the most devastating result of anorexia is death.

Complications of Bulimia

While it is commonly thought that the medical problems resulting from bulimia are not as severe as those resulting from anorexia, the complications are numerous and gravely serious. The medical problems associated with bulimia include tooth erosion, cavities, and gum problems due to the acid in vomit. Abdominal bloating is common in bulimic individuals. The purging process can leave a person dehydrated and with very low potassium levels which can cause weakness and paralysis. Some of the more severe problems a bulimic can suffer include reproductive problems and heart damage, due to the lack of minerals in the body.

Ways to Help Someone with an Eating Disorder

The best course of action for a person who suspects they know someone with an eating disorder is to be patient, supportive, and not judge the individual. Learn what you can about the problem by consulting an eating disorder clinic or counseling center (common on college campuses), and offer to help the ill person seek professional help.

Medical treatment is often necessary for eating disorders. The best and most successful treatment is a combination of counseling, family therapy, cognitive behavior therapy, nutritional therapy, support groups, and drug therapy. Treatment many times includes a hospital stay and is usually resisted by the patient. Support for the anorexic or bulimic person by friends and family and the realization of the severity of the problem is critical to successful treatment of the illness.

References

Donatelle, R.J. & L.G. Davis. *Access to Health*. 4th ed. Boston, MA: Allyn and Bacon, 1996.

Floyd, P.A., et al. *Personal Health: Perspectives & Lifestyles*. 2d ed., Englewood, CO: Morton Publishing Company, 1998.

I Have Won

One Woman's Recovery
from Binge Eating Disorder

It was a constant nagging voice in my mind, whispering promises of protection, comfort and a life of numbness. I didn't realize it was my enemy, disguised as a savior. This is what my eating disorder was to me. I have been struggling with Binge Eating Disorder for eight years and after a year of therapy I am learning how to tell that voice to go away and to love, trust and respect myself and my values.

I have countless memories of daytime binges when my roommates were in class, even digging through the trash to retrieve a half-eaten candy bar or piece of cake. I withdrew from my friends, missed out on beach parties, and felt lonely, scared and completely out of control every waking moment of the day. I became deeply depressed and couldn't face emotional issues that had been with me for a long time. That voice gave soothing promises of a way out, a way to forget, an excuse for any failures or disappointments, and a way to slowly…die.

My friends and family were aware there was a problem but I spent years denying the truth. I would tell them I just loved to eat and I just needed to start exercising more. All the while my weight kept slowly growing. I would think constantly about changing, going on a diet, but the diet day would come and I couldn't do it, so I would retreat to the voice and let it take charge. I finally accepted that I had a problem when I was in school completing a Master's Degree in Counseling. I had to constantly analyze myself and my life for projects and papers and could no longer deny the issues at hand.

I entered into therapy and honestly wasn't prepared for the difficulty that lay ahead. I had to confront my demons, that voice, examine every horrible issue that I had suppressed and once again learn how to live life. I learned that I can do other things when I find myself in front of the refrigerator and I am not physically hungry. I can take walks, call my husband, or put together a puzzle. I also had to relearn my body's signals for hunger and fullness and to trust that my body will tell me what I need and when I need it.

Although still in recovery, I can clearly see how far I've come, and I can see the light at the end of the tunnel. I now spend time speaking about eating disorders and volunteering at the Massachusetts Eating Disorder Association. I want people to know that there is hope and that recovery is possible. The voice no longer whispers to me; I now shout at it, "I don't need you anymore. I love myself. I have won!"

by Cathy King, M.S.

A special thanks
to the Massachusetts Eating Disorder Association

Courtesy of the Massachusetts Eating Disorder Association.

Hales, Dianne. *An Invitation to Health*. 8th ed. New York, NY: Brooks/Cole Publishing Company, 1999.

Hoeger, Werner, and Sharon Hoeger. *Principle and Labs for Fitness and Wellness*. 5th ed. Englewood, CO: Morton Publishing Company, 1999.

Hyman, B., et al. *Fitness for Living*. Dubuque, Iowa: Kendall/Hunt Publishing Company, 1999.

Jeffrey, D.B. & R.C. Katz. *Take It Off and Keep It Off: A Behavioral Program for Weight Loss and Healthy Living*. Englewood Cliffs, NJ: Prentice-Hall, 1977.

Powers, S.K. & S.L. Todd. *Total Fitness*. Boston, MA: Allyn and Bacon, 1996.

Prentice, William, E. *Fitness and Wellness for Life*. 6th ed., New York, NY: WCB McGraw-Hill, 1999.

Pruitt, B.E. & J. Stein. *HealthStyles*. 2d ed., Boston, MA: Allyn and Bacon, 1999.

Robbins, Gwen, et al. *A Wellness Way of Life*. 4th ed. New York, NY: WCB McGraw-Hill, 1999.

Rosato, Frank. *Fitness for Wellness.* 3d ed. Minneapolis, MN: West Publishing, 1994.

Scanlon, D. & L. Strauss. *Diets That Work: For Weight Control or Medical Needs.* Los Angeles, CA: Lowell House, 1991.

Dietary Guidelines. Ganesa. http://www.ganesa.com/food/foodpyramid.gif

Nutrition Guidelines. Health Depot. http://www.healthdepot.com

Contacts

American Dietetics Association
http://www.eatright.org

Food and Nutrition Center of the U.S.D.A.
http://www.nal.usda.gov/fnic

General Nutrition Site
http://www.healthy.net/index.html

National Association of Anorexia Nervosa and Associated Disorders
http://www.injersey.com/Living/Health/anad.index.html

Eating Disorder Awareness Prevention
http://members.aol.com/edapinc/home.html

American Anorexia/Bulimia Association, Inc.
http://www.members.aol.com/amanbu/index/html

National Eating Disorder Organization
665 South Yale Ave.
Tulsa, OK. 74136
(918)481-4044

Healthfinder
http://www.healthfinder.gov

National Institutes of Health
http://www.nih.gov/health

Mayo Clinic Health Informatin
http://www.mayo.ivi.com

CNNs Health Report
http://www.cnn.com/HEALTH

Activities

In-Class Activities
    Fatty Boom-Ba-Latty
    Hey Good Lookin', What's Cookin'?

Out-of-Class Activities (Notebook)

U.S. RDA Information Sheet	(1 point)
Eating and Emotions	(1 point)
Mirror, Mirror on the Wall	(1 point)
Eating Disorders: Anorexia Nervosa	(2 points)
Eating Disorders: Bulimia Nervosa	(2 points)
Food Processor	(5 points)

■ Fatty Boom-Ba-Latty

Directions: For each item below, place an X in the box indicating which food you think contains more fat.

☐ 2 slices cheese pizza   ☐ 1 peanut butter and jelly sandwich

☐ 1 fish sandwich   ☐ 1 roasted pork chop

☐ 1 cup spaghetti and meatballs   ☐ 10 french fries

☐ 1 small taco   ☐ 10 baked potatoes

☐ 3 oz. fish sticks   ☐ 1/2 croissant

☐ 2 sausage links   ☐ 2 English muffins

☐ 1 regular cheeseburger   ☐ 1/2 cup canned pudding

☐ 3 oz. sirloin steak   ☐ 10 oz. vanilla milkshake

☐ 6 pancakes   ☐ 1 cup macaroni and cheese

☐ 1 cinnamon sweet roll   ☐ 10 slices bread

☐ 2 cups lowfat yogurt   ☐ 1 oz. tortilla chips

☐ 1 tablespoon mayonnaise   ☐ 1 cup unbuttered popcorn

■ Hey Good Lookin', What's Cookin'?

Concept/Description: Society has conditioned people, especially females, to believe that thin is beautiful.

Objective: To recognize the effect the media has had on body image and self-concept.

Materials: Hey, Baby…
Magazine ads of attractive models advertising any product
Pens or pencils

Directions:
1. Divide the class into pairs and give each pair a magazine ad showing an attractive model.
2. Ask pairs to look at the ad and fill in the Hey, Baby… worksheet.
3. When all have finished analyzing their ads, have pairs show their ads and briefly describe their findings.
4. Ask students if they feel these images are realistic and whether this could contribute to eating disorders. Discuss.
5. Although most anorexics and bulimics are girls, some are boys. Ask the class why they feel there are more girls than boys suffering from eating disorders. Discuss.

Variations:
1. Videotape TV commercials of "beautiful people" and analyze them as a class.
2. Have students make up their own commercials emphasizing the use of "beautiful people" to advertise anything from automobiles to food.
3. Have students videotape public service announcements highlighting the dangers of eating disorders. Play them for the class.

■ Hey, Baby...

Directions: Analyze the advertisement given to you and answer the questions.

1. Describe the people shown in your advertisement.

2. What product is being advertised?

3. Is the emphasis in your ad on the product or the people?

4. Why do you think the advertiser used those particular people in the ad? What does the ad seem to imply?

5. Do you think the people in the ad represent typical Americans? Why or why not?

6. Do you think people tend to compare themselves to the images the media portrays?

7. How can associating beautiful people with products help to sell the products?

8. Do you think the media has contributed to some people having eating disorders? Why or why not? Explain.

■ U.S. RDA Information Sheet

Many nutrients on a food label are listed as a percentage of the U.S. Recommended Daily Allowances. The U.S. RDA are the amount of nutrients needed each day by most healthy people.

The following are U.S. RDA for these nutrients:

Protein	45 g
Vitamin A	5000 IU
Vitamin C	60 mg
Thiamin	1.5 mg
Riboflavin	1.7 mg
Niacin	20 mg
Calcium	1000 mg
Iron	18 mg

Directions: Look at the food label below and answer the questions.

TONS-O-BRAN CEREAL

Percentages of U.S. Recommended Daily Allowances

Protein	5%
Vitamin A	25%
Vitamin C	4%
Thiamine	25%
Riboflavin	25%
Calcium	2%
Iron	45%
Vitamin D	10%

How many bowls of cereal would you have to eat to meet the U.S. RDA for:

1. Vitamin A? _____

2. Protein? _____

3. Calcium? _____

What would be a better way to meet the U.S. RDA? Explain.

■ **Eating and Emotions**

Hunger, according to scientists, is physiological, a sensation that occurs when the blood sugar begins to drop and the stomach contracts. But we are all aware that many people eat for emotional reasons as well. Try the quiz below to give you some idea of how well attuned you are to your own habits and how your emotions influence your eating habits.

Directions: Use the following guidelines to give yourself a score of 0–8 for each item:

    8   Very often—almost every other day
    6   Often—one to three times a week
    4   Occasionally—two to three times a month
    2   Rarely—once every month to three months
    0   Never

1. I eat foods that I know aren't nutritious. _____
2. I eat meals or heavy snacks after 7 at night. _____
3. I'm afraid I'll gain weight. _____
4. I eat when I'm not hungry. _____
5. I eat foods my parents don't want me to eat. _____
6. I'm self-conscious about how I look. _____
7. When I'm bored or depressed, I eat a lot. _____
8. I go on eating binges. _____
9. I eat until I'm uncomfortable. _____
10. I hide foods or sneak them. _____
11. I eat because I feel "who cares?" _____
12. I drink alcoholic beverages. _____
13. I have uncontrollable urges of hunger. _____
14. Feelings of anger or hostility overwhelm me. _____
15. I indulge in sweets. _____
16. I eat when I'm tired or overtired. _____
17. I like to eat alone. _____
18. I use appetite suppressants. _____
19. My parents made sweets available or used them for rewards. _____
20. I eat and run. _____
21. I don't have respect for myself and my body. _____
22. I feel rushed or hurried. _____
23. I have a snack or meal an hour before I go to bed. _____
24. I crave sweet foods. _____
25. When I eat with other people, I feel self-conscious. _____
26. I gulp my food. _____
27. I wish I looked like someone else. _____
28. I eat or drink in secret. _____
29. I feel as if I'm in the middle of a struggle. _____
30. I eat when I can't sleep. _____

From *Just for the Health of It: Unit 2, Diet and Nutrition Activities* by Patricia Rizzo Toner. Copyright © 1993. Reprinted by permission of Center for Applied Research in Education/Prentice Hall Direct.

■ Scoring for Eating and Emotions

What your score means:

120 and below:	Good relationship with your body; sensitive to physical needs
120-160:	Average range for normally healthy people
161-190:	Eating is based too much on emotional needs.
191 and above:	Excessive emotional interference in eating habits.

When emotions lead to poor nutritional habits, it can affect the normal functioning of the body. This, in turn, can make us feel listless. Bingeing, gorging, eating at the wrong time, or constant snacking can result in bloating and eventually obesity. Eating too fast or too much can interfere with the digestive system's ability to use nutrients properly.

Answer the Following Questions:

1. Into which category does your score place you?

2. Are you happy or unhappy with your eating habits? Explain.

3. What can you do to improve your eating habits? (List at least three suggestions.)

■ Mirror, Mirror on the Wall

Directions: How you feel about your body can affect your self-confidence and attitude toward life. Rank each body part according to the way you perceive yourself, then add up your score below.

	Very Satisfied (4)	Satisfied (3)	Dissatisfied (2)	Very Unhappy (1)
Height				
Weight				
Thighs				
Calves				
Hips				
Arms				
Shoulders				
Skin				
Hair				
Eyes				
Ears				
Nose				
Mouth				
Stomach				

How do you rate yourself?   44-56 You are very satisfied
                            34-43 You are satisfied
                            24-33 You are somewhat dissatisfied.
                            14-23 Think positive, you probably look better than you think!

From *Just for the Health of It: Unit 5, Stress Management and Self-Esteem Activities* by Patricia Rizzo Toner.
Copyright © 1993. Reprinted by permission of Center for Applied Research in Education/Prentice Hall Direct.

■ Eating Disorders: Anorexia Nervosa

Directions: Research the eating disorder Anorexia Nervosa and answer the questions.

1. What is Anorexia Nervosa?

2. What are some of the possible causes?

3. What are the signs and symptoms?

4. What are the health risks?

5. Where, in your community, can you get help for eating disorders?

From *Just for the Health of It: Unit 2, Diet and Nutrition Activities* by Patricia Rizzo Toner. Copyright © 1993. Reprinted by permission of Center for Applied Research in Education/Prentice Hall Direct.

■ Eating Disorders: Bulimia

Directions: Research the eating disorder Bulimia and answer the questions.

1. What is Bulimia?

2. What are some of the possible causes?

3. What are the signs and symptoms?

4. What are the health risks?

5. Where, in your community, can you get help for eating disorders?

■ Food Processor Optional Notebook Assignment

Health & Fitness
5 points

Record all that you eat for three days. Include at least one weekend day and one weekday for a total of three days. Use as much detail as possible, including amount and type of food. The more accurate your record, the more accurate your analysis will be. Be specific!

Example: 1 cup of fruity pebbles
                      1 cup of 1% milk
                      1 small package of peanut M&M's (6 oz.)
                      1 large coffee black (8 oz.)

Take your food list, and go to 150 READ bldg. computer lab. **Bring your student ID and get a lab log-on ID and password if you don't already have one. This will take an extra 10–15 minutes.** Secure a food processor instruction sheet from the shelves and follow the directions. (You will be working on a Mac.) Input all your food from the 3 days together. No need to separate out the days. You may need to make some substitutions, however the food inventory list has much to choose from. If you have problems, ask the personnel behind the help desk. Print out *everything*—that should be ***4 print-outs** if you followed the directions completely*. Please staple the 4 papers together in the order that you ran them off. Good Luck!

Note: Most people overestimate their activity level and underestimate their food intake. Be as accurate as possible! Most of us probably fall into moderate activity level.

If you have problems finding a food item, backspace several times, then double check to see that you are spelling the item correctly. Sometimes you will find carrots where you couldn't find carrot—change plural to singular and vice-versa. Finally, think of other names—such as toaster pastries instead of pop-tarts.

Ask for help at the help desk if need be!

*Remember to eat as normally as you can!

Appendix

Health & Fitness Notebook

Be certain to complete each activity for full credit.

5 Point Activities

Cardiovascular and Muscular Fitness

Developing an exercise program for cardiorespiratory endurance—Complete the assignment on pg. _55._

Diseases

Develop Family Tree—In order to do this project you must first research your family history. You may do an oral history or written correspondence with a family member or you may research old records. Identify your source or sources of information. Record diseases and afflictions of all known family members through your great-grandparents. Pay particular attention to genetic disorders and the age of onset. Have you inherited cardiac risk factors? Common factors to consider are family history of heart disease, diabetes, high blood pressure, high cholesterol and some forms of cancer. What, if any, diseases are you at risk for due to your family history? What can you do now to have an impact on your long-term health for the future? How do you intend to avoid becoming "at-risk" in the future? Please detail your family history in the first paragraph. In the second paragraph relate how you can live your lifestyle now to best insure you have a long and healthy life.

Nutrition

Food Processor—Write down three days worth of food/drink in great detail (e.g. 1 cup of fruity pebbles with ½ cup of skim milk, 6 oz. orange juice, 2 oz. plain M&Ms) before you go to Read 150, Blocker, Student Computing Center or West Campus to do the assignment. Be sure to include at least one weekend day and one weekday, not all three weekdays. Eat as normally as you can! You need to have a labs access account number if you do not already have one (e.g. to check e-mail). Bring your ID with you to which ever computing center you choose to use. Pick up the instructions from the help desk, labeled "The Food Processor". Follow the instructions and you will have four printouts. Allow approximately one hour to complete this assignment.

2 Point Activities

Defining Health

Stress Journal—Follow the form on pg. _25_

Have a Laugh—Complete the form on pg. _27_

Cardiovascular and Muscular Fitness

Assessing your current level of muscular endurance—Complete the form on pg. ___

Assessing your current level of muscular strength—Complete the form on pg. _57_

Hypokinetic Conditions

AHA Health Risk Awareness (http://www.americanheart.org/risk/quiz.html)—Go to the website, complete the questionnaire and print out your results. Turn in your answers to the questions along with the result printout for credit.

Self-Assessment of Cardiovascular Fitness—Complete the form on pg. _73_

Healthy Back Test—Complete the form on pg. _75_

Body Fat Percentage (skin calipers or water weighing)—Performed by a licensed individual, turn in actual results from test.

Diseases

Blood Glucose Level—Performed by a licensed individual, turn in actual results from test.

Nutrition

Cholesterol Levels measured—Performed by a licensed individual, turn in actual results from test.

Eating Disorders: Anorexia Nervosa—Complete the form on pg. _191_

Eating Disorders: Bulimia Nervosa—Complete the form on pg. _193_

1 Point Activities

Defining Health

What's My Line—Complete the assignment on pg. 21

I Like That—Complete the form on pg. 23

College Schedule of Recent Experience—Complete the form on pg. 29

Cardiovascular and Muscular Fitness

Par-Q and you—Complete the form on pg. 49

Calculating your activity index—Complete the form on pg. 51

Determine an accurate heart rate—Complete the form on pg. 53

Hypokinetic Conditions

Blood Pressure Reading—Performed by a licensed individual, turn in actual results from test.

Safety Awareness

Checklist of rape prevention strategies—Complete the form on pg. 85

Sexuality

What Is Your Risk of Contracting a Sexually Transmitted Infection?—Complete the form on pg. 111

STD Risk Profiler (http://www.unspeakable.com/nph-survey.cgi?tag=risk)—Go to the website, complete the questionnaire and print out your results. Turn in your answers to the questions along with the result printout for credit.

STD Quiz (http://www.unspeakable.com/nph-survey.cgi?tag=std)—Go to the website, complete the questionnaire and print out your results. Turn in your answers to the questions along with the result printout for credit.

STI Attitudes—Complete the form on pg. 117. Be sure to tally up your score for credit. The range for scores is 27-135.

Successful Contraception Questionnaire (http://www.arhp.org/success/index.html)—Go to the website, complete the questionnaire and print out your results. Turn in your answers to the questions along with the result printout for credit.

Diseases

Check your asthma "I.Q."—Complete the form on pg. 135

Could you have diabetes and not know it?—Complete the form on pg. 137

Drugs

Self-survey: Are you addicted to nicotine?—Complete the form on pg. 169

What kind of drinker are you?—Complete the form on pg. 171

Nutrition

U.S. RDA Information Sheet—Complete the form on pg. _185_

Eating and Emotions—Complete the form on pg. _187_

Mirror, Mirror on the Wall—Complete the form on pg. _189_

Health & Fitness Notebook Tally Sheet

NAME _____   SECTION _____

Instructions: Please place this at the front of your notebook and mark all of the activities that you completed.

5 Point Activities
Cardiovascular and Muscular Fitness
    Developing an exercise program for cardiorespiratory endurance   _____
Nutrition
    Food Processor   _____
Diseases
    Develop Family Tree   _____

2 Point Activities
Defining Health
    Stress Journal   _____
    Have a laugh   _____
Cardiovascular and Muscular Fitness
    Assessing your current level of muscular endurance   _____
    Assessing your current level of muscular strength   _____
Hypokinetic Conditions
    AHA Health Risk Awareness (internet)   _____
    Self-Assessment of Cardiovascular Fitness   _____
    Healthy Back Test   _____
    Body Fat Percentage (skin calipers or water weighing)   _____
Diseases
    Blood Glucose Level   _____
Nutrition
    Cholesterol Levels measured   _____
    Eating Disorders: Anorexia Nervosa   _____
    Eating Disorders: Bulimia Nervosa   _____

1 Point Activities
Defining Health
    What's My Line   _____
    I Like That   _____
    College Schedule of Recent Experience   _____
Cardiovascular and Muscular Fitness
    Par-Q and you   _____
    Calculating your activity index   _____
    Determine an accurate heart rate   _____

Hypokinetic Conditions

Blood Pressure Reading   _____

Safety Awareness

Checklist of rape prevention strategies   _____

Sexuality

What Is Your Risk of Contracting a Sexually Transmitted Infection?   _____

STD Risk Profiler (internet)   _____

STD Quiz (internet)   _____

STI Attitudes   _____

Successful Contraception Questionnaire (internet)   _____

Diseases

Check your asthma "I.Q."   _____

Could you have diabetes and not know it?   _____

Drugs

What kind of drinker are you?   _____

Self-Survey: Are you addicted to nicotine?   _____

Nutrition

U.S. RDA Information Sheet   _____

Eating and Emotions   _____

Mirror, Mirror on the Wall   _____

TOTAL   _____

Glossary

Abortion—any expulsion from the uterus of a fetus before it is able to survive.

Abstinence—to voluntarily do without.

Accident—that occurrence in a sequence of events which produces unintended injury, death, or property damage.

Acquired immune deficiency syndrome—a reliably diagnosed disease that is at least moderately indicative of an underlying cellular immune deficiency, for example Kaposi's sarcoma in a patient aged less than sixty years or opportunistic infection where there is no known underlying cause of cellular immune deficiency nor any other cause of reduced resistance reported to be associated with the disease.

Activity Nervosa—a condition where the individual suffers from an ever-present compulsion to exercise, regardless of illness or injury.

Adenosine triphosphate (ATP)—high energy compound formed from oxidation of fat and carbohydrate and used as an energy supply.

Adoption—to take legally into one's own family and raise as one's own child.

Aerobic—means "in the presence of oxygen," and is used synonymously with cardiovascular.

Alcohol Poisoning—an overdose of alcohol, which may lead to death.

Alcoholism—is a chronic progressive disease that includes a strong need to drink alcohol despite the negative consequences.

Alveoli—tiny air sacs in the lungs through whose walls gases such as oxygen and carbon dioxide diffuse in and out of blood.

Amino acid—organic compounds containing carbon, hydrogen, nitrogen, and oxygen. They are the building blocks of protein.

Amphetamines—drugs that stimulate the nervous system.

Anaerobic—occurring in the absence of oxygen.

Anemia—a condition in which the blood is low in red cells or in hemoglobin, resulting in paleness and weakness.

Angina pectoris—insufficient blood flow to the heart muscle that results in severe chest and arm pain.

Anorexia Nervosa—a state of starvation and emaciation usually resulting from severe dieting and excessive exercise.

Antioxidants—compounds that come to the aid of every cell in the body facing an ongoing barrage of damage resulting from daily oxygen exposure, environmental pollution, chemicals and pesticides, additives in processed foods, stress hormones, and sun radiation.

Anus—is the opening located just behind the perineum at the lower end of the alimentary canal that allows for elimination of solid waste.

Aorta—the large artery that receives blood from the left ventricle and distributes it to the body.

Arrhythmia—an irregularity in the rhythm of the heartbeat that often precedes a heart attack.

Arteriosclerosis—hardening of the arteries.

Asthma—a respiratory disorder which involves difficulty breathing, wheezing and/or coughing due to the constriction of the bronchial tubes.

Asymptomatic—without symptoms.

Atherosclerosis—long-term buildup of fatty deposits and other substances such as cholesterol, cellular waste products, calcium and fibrin on the interior walls of arteries.

Atria—the two upper chambers of the heart in which blood collects before passing to the ventricles.

BAC—Blood Alcohol Concentration; the ratio of alcohol measured in the blood to total blood volume.

Bacteria—microorganisms which have no chlorophyll and multiply by simple division: some bacteria cause diseases, but others are necessary for fermentation.

Barbiturates—depressants used to induce sleep and relaxation.

Benign—non-invasive, non-cancerous (of a growth). Describes a condition or illness which is not serious and does not usually have harmful consequences.

Binge drinking—consuming five or more alcoholic beverages in one sitting for men, four for women.

Bingeing—consuming an excessive amount of food in a short period of time.

Blackout—individual has amnesia about events after drinking though there was no loss of consciousness.

Blood pressure—the force exerted by the blood on the walls of the blood vessels; 120/80 is considered average.

Body composition—measures percentage of body fat in relation to their percentage of lean body mass (muscle, bone and internal organs.)

Breast—the mammary gland.

Bulimia Nervosa—a process of bingeing and purging.

Caffeine—mild stimulant found in cola, coffee, chocolate.

Cancer—a general term which covers any malignant growth in any part of the body. The growth is purposeless, parasitic and flourishes at the expense of the human host.

Cancer—is characterized by the spread of abnormal cells that serve no useful purpose.

Carbohydrates—the body's main source of fuel. Between 55–60% of an individual's diet should be composed of carbohydrates.

Carbon Monoxide—odorless, tasteless gas that is highly toxic and contains carcinogens.

Carcinoma—any of several kinds of epithelial cancer.

Cardiovascular—pertaining to the heart and blood vessels.

Cardiovascular endurance—the ability of the body to perform prolonged, large-muscle, dynamic exercise at moderate-to-high levels of intensity. In order for this process to occur, the heart, lungs, and blood vessels must deliver oxygen to working muscles and the body's metabolic system must use oxygen to process fuels for sustained activity.

Cardiovascular exercise—when performed within certain guidelines, develops higher levels of cardiovascular endurance by improving the efficiency and strength of the cardiovascular system. Cardiovascular exercise, uses large muscle groups in a continuous, rhythmic nature for an extended period of time.

Cervix—the neck of the uterus.

Cesarean section—delivery of the fetus through an abdominal incision.

Chemotherapy—use of a specific chemical agent to arrest the progress of, or eradicate, disease in the body without causing irreversible injury to healthy tissues.

Chlamydia—is a sexually transmitted infection caused by bacteria-like intracellular parasite called Chlamydia trachomati which can infect humans and birds.

Cholesterol—a crystalline substance of a fatty nature found in the brain, nerves, liver, blood and bile. It is not easily soluble and may crystallize in the gallbladder and along arterial walls.

Clitoral hood—consists of inner lips, which join to form a soft fold of skin, or hood, covering and connecting to the clitoris.

Clitoris—a small erectile organ of the female genitalia.

Cocaine—psychoactive substance found in the leaves of the coca plant; stimulant.

Codeine—narcotic commonly found in cough suppressant.

Cold—viral infection of the respiratory tract, causing congestion, sneezing, sore throat, coughing and a low-grade fever.

Colon—the large bowel extending from the cecum to the rectum.

Coma—deep, prolonged unconsciousness caused by injury or disease.

Communicable—transmissible directly or indirectly from one person to another.

Complex carbohydrates—provide the body with a steady source of energy for hours. The best sources of complex carbohydrates are breads, cereals, pastas, and grains.

Conception—the creation of a state of pregnancy; impregnation of the ovum by the sperm.

Condom—(male) a rubber sheath used as a male contraceptive. (Female) a sheath, made of latex, placed into the vagina before sexual intercourse. These condoms help protect both partners against sexually transmitted infection.

Coronary arteries—two arteries branching from the aorta that provide blood to the heart muscle.

Cowper's glands—responsible for depositing a lubricant fluid in the semen to help with sperm motility.

Depo-Provera—a hormone shot injected into the arm or buttocks every twelve weeks.

Depressants—category of drugs that depress the nervous system.

Depression—a hollow or low place.

Diabetes—the result of insufficient insulin production or the body's inability to utilize insulin readily produced by the pancreas.

Diaphragm—a rubber cap which encircles the cervix to act as a contraceptive. It should be used with a spermicidal jelly or cream.

Diastolic blood pressure—the lowest arterial pressure attained during the heart cycle.

Dietary fiber (roughage or bulk)—a type of complex carbohydrate that is present mainly in leaves, roots, skins and seeds. Dietary fiber is the part of the plant that is not digested in the small intestine, and it helps decrease the risk of cardiovascular disease, cancer, and may lower an individual's risk of coronary heart.

Disease—any deviation from or interruption of the normal structure and function of any part of the body. It is manifested by a characteristic set of signs and symptoms and in most instances the origin, route of transmission and prognosis is known.

Distress—negative stress. It is a physically and mentally damaging response to the demands placed upon the body.

Ecstsy—a drug that is chemically similar to mescaline and methamphetamines.

Ejaculation—the sudden emission of semen from the erect penis at the moment of male orgasm.

Epididymis—a small oblong body attached to the posterior surface of the testes. Mature sperm are stored in the epididymis until they are released during ejaculation.

Epithelium—cellular tissue covering external body surfaces or lining internal surfaces.

Essential amino acid—amino acids that the body cannot produce, thus they must be supplied through an individual's diet.

Estrogen—a generic term referring to ovarian hormones.

Ethyl alcohol—a colorless liquid that depresses the nervous system. Made by the fermentation process and found in alcohol.

ETS—Environmental Tobacco Smoke; second hand smoke inhaled by the non-smoker.

Eustress—a positive stress that produces a state of well-being.

Exercise prescription—individualization of an exercise program on the basis of the exercise duration, frequency, intensity, and mode.

Exercise stress test—a test that involves analysis of the changes in electrical activity in the heart from an electrocardiogram taken during exercise.

Fallopian tubes—these tubes extend from beside the ovaries to the uterus and transport developed ovum. Fertilization usually takes place within the fallopian tubes.

Fats—the body's primary source of energy. Fat has many essential functions, including: providing the body with stored energy, insulating the body to preserve body heat, contributing to cellular structure, and protecting vital organs by absorbing shock.

Fat-soluble vitamins—vitamins transported by the body's fat cells and by the liver. They include vitamins A, E, D, and K.

Fear of obesity—an over-concern with thinness.

Fertilization—the impregnation of an ovum by a sperm.

Fetal Alcohol Syndrome—a group of physical and behavioral defects in a newborn causes by the mother's alcohol use during pregnancy.

Fibrin—insoluble blood protein formed in blood clots.

Foreskin—the prepuce or skin covering the glans penis.

Gastrointestinal—pertaining to the stomach and intestine.

GHB—Gamma Hydroxybutrate—a fast acting, powerful drug that depresses the nervous system.

Glucose—a simple sugar that circulates in the blood and can be used by cells to fuel ATP production.

Glycogen—a complex carbohydrate stored principally in the liver and skeletal muscles that is the major fuel source during most forms of intense exercise.

Gonorrhea—is a sexually transmitted infection caused by the bacteria called Neisseria gonorrhea.

Hallucinogens—drugs that affect perception, sensation and awareness.

Hazard—conditions or set of conditions which have the potential to produce injury and/or property damage.

Health—a state of complete physical, mental, and social well-being and not merely the absence of disease or infirmity.

Heart attack—when an artery that provides the heart muscle with oxygen becomes blocked or flow is decreased.

Hepatitis—inflammation of the liver in response to toxins or infective agents.

Heroin—a very strong narcotic.

Herpes—a chronic, lifelong viral sexually transmitted infection that can cause small blisters on the skin and mucous membranes.

High-density lipoprotein—a plasma protein relatively high in protein, low in cholesterol. HDL help eliminate cholesterol from the body.

Human chorionic gonadotrophin (HCG)—a hormone arising from the placenta. The presence of HCG in urine is detectable in an early morning specimen of urine from the sixth week of pregnancy.

Human immunodeficiency virus—is a retrovirus that infects human T cells and is believed to cause acquired immune deficiency syndrome.

Human papilloma viruses—are the viruses that cause genital warts and have a high correlation with cervical cancer.

Hymen—the thin mucous membrane that closes part or sometimes all of the opening of the vagina.

Hypertension—abnormally high blood pressure.

Hypokinetic—too little activity.

Immunotherapy—any treatment used to produce immunity.

Implantation—the insertion of living cells or solid materials into the tissues, e.g. implantation of the fertilized ovum into the endometrium.

Influenza—an acute, contagious viral disease, characterized by inflammation of the respiratory tract, fever and muscular pain.

Inhalants—chemicals that produce vapors having psychoactive effects.

Insoluble fiber—dietary fiber which does not dissolve easily in water; therefore, it cannot be digested by the body.

Insomnia—abnormal inability to sleep.

Intoxication—a transient state of physical and mental disruption due to the presence of a toxic substance such as alcohol.

Intrauterine device—a small plastic device that is inserted into the uterus to impede conception or prevent implantation of a fertilized egg.

Irritable bowel syndrome—unusual motility of both small and large bowel which produces discomfort and intermittent pain, for which no organic cause can be found.

Ischemia—reduced blood flow.

Labia majora—two longitudinal folds of skin that extend on both sides of the vulva and serve as protection for the inner parts of the vulva.

Labia minora—the delicate inner folds of skin that enclose the urethral opening and the vagina.

Lactic acid—a metabolic acid resulting from the metabolism of glucose and glycogen. Accumulation will produce fatigue.

Lactovegetarians—individuals that eat dairy products, fruits, and vegetables but do not consume any other animal products (meat, poultry, fish, or eggs.)

Legume—a pod, such as that of a pea or bean that splits into two halves with the seeds attached to one of the halves.

Leukemia—a disease characterized by an abnormal increase in the number of leukocytes.

Leukoplakia—pre-cancerous condition that produces thick, rough, white patches on the gums, tongue and inner cheek.

Lice—plural form of louse. Small, wingless parasite found on humans and some animals.

Low-density lipoproteins—are major cholesterol carriers that bind to receptors in various tissues, including liver, muscle and arteries. High levels of LDL are likely to lead to atherosclerosis.

LSD—Lysergic Acid Diethylamide; hallucinogenic drug that distorts reality.

Lung—either of the two spongelike breathing organs in the thorax of vertebrates.

Lymphoma—any of a group of diseases resulting from the proliferation of malignant lymphoid cells.

Macrominerals—the seven minerals the body needs in relatively large quantities (100 mg. or more each day.)

Macronutrients—provide energy in the form of calories. They include carbohydrates, fats, and proteins.

Malignant—virulent and dangerous; that which is likely to have a fatal termination.

Marijuana—from the cannabis sativa plant where the leaves and stems are dried and rolled into cigarettes.

Maximal oxygen consumption—(VO_{2max}) the highest rate of oxygen consumption an individual is capable of during maximum physical effort. Measured in ml/kg/min.

Melanoma—a tumor arising from the pigment-producing cells of the deeper layers in the skin.

Menstruation—the flow of blood from the uterus once a month in the female. It commences about the age of thirteen years and ceases at about forty-five years of age.

Metabolism—the sum of all the vital processes by which food energy and nutrients are made available to and used by the body.

Microminerals—mineral that are essential to healthy living. They are needed in small quantities (less than 100 mg. per day.)

Micronutrients—regulate many bodily functions such as, metabolism, growth, and development. They include vitamins and minerals.

Minerals—inorganic substances that are critical to many enzyme functions in the body.

Mononucleosis—a self-limiting viral infection causing a sore throat, fatigue, fever and possible spleen enlargement.

Monounsaturated fats—fats found in foods such as olives, peanuts, and canola oil, peanut oil, and olive oil.

Mons pubis—the soft fatty tissue covering the pubic symphysis on the female genitalia.

Morphine—narcotic used for quick pain relief.

Myocardial infarct—heart attack.

Narcotic—drugs used to relieve pain.

Nicotine—highly addictive compound that is extremely poisonous.

Non-essential amino acids—amino acids that are manufactured in the body if food proteins in a person's diet provide enough nitrogen.

Norplant—consists of six small capsules placed under the skin which constantly release small amounts of the hormone progestin.

Obesity—the deposition of excessive fat around the body, particularly in the subcutaneous tissue.

Occlusion—the closure of an opening, especially of ducts or blood vessels.

Occupational illness—conditions caused by repeated exposure associated with employment.

Opium—the base substance for all narcotics.

Oral—pertaining to the mouth.

Oral contraceptive (the pill)—a prescription medication containing the hormones estrogen and/or progestin.

Osteoporosis—a disease characterized by a loss of bone density.

Ovary—female reproductive gland where eggs are produced and released usually once a month.

Over-training—a condition caused by training too much or too intensely.

Ovolactovegetarians—a type of vegetarian that eats eggs as well as dairy products, fruits, and vegetables, but does not consume meat, poultry, and or fish.

Parasite—one who lives at others' expense without making any useful return.

Parent—a person in relation to his or her offspring; a mother or father.

PCP—Phencyclidine hydrochloride; hallucinogenic drug which blocks pain and produces numbness.

Penis—the male organ through which semen and urine pass and has three main sections: the root, shaft and glans penis.

Perineum—the smooth skin located between the labia minora and the anus.

Peripheral vascular disease—any abnormal condition arising in the blood vessels outside the heart, the main one being atherosclerosis, which can lead to thrombosis and occlusion of the vessel resulting in gangrene.

Pernicious—causing great injury or destruction.

Physical fitness—the ability of the body to respond or adapt to the demands and stress of physical effort.

Polyunsaturated fats—fats found in margarine, pecans, corn oil, cottonseed oil, sunflower oil, and soybean oil.

Pregnancy—being with child, e.g. gestation from last menstrual period to delivery, normally 40 weeks or 280 days.

Prostate—a small gland at the base of the male bladder and surrounding the urethra.

Protein—essential "building blocks" of the body. They are needed for the growth, maintenance, and repair of all body tissues.

Psychoactive drugs—any agent that has the ability to alter moods, behavior and perception.

Pubic—in the region of the genitals.

Pulmonary circulation—the part of the circulatory system that moves blood between the heart and the lungs.

Purging—self-induced vomiting or elimination of food.

Ratings of perceived exertion—a system of monitoring exercise intensity based on assigning a number to the subjective perception of target intensity.

Rectum—the lowest or last segment of the large intestine.

Respiratory system—the lungs, air passages, and breathing muscles which supplies oxygen and removes carbon dioxide from the body by way of the circulatory system.

Reye's syndrome—consists of cerebral edema without cellular infiltration. The age range of recorded cases is two months to fifteen years of age. Presents with vomiting, lethargy, confusion, rapid heartbeat and respiration. May progress into a coma. There is an association with aspirin administration and viral infections.

Risk—the probability that a hazard will be activated and produce injury and/or property damage.

Rohypnol—a drug prescribed for sleep disorders; potent tranquilizer; "date rape drug."

Sarcoma—malignant growth of the connective tissue including muscles and bones.

Saturated fats—fats found primarily in animal products such as meats, lard, cream, butter, cheese, and whole milk.

Scabies—a highly contagious, itching skin disease caused by a mite that burrows under the skin to lay its eggs.

Scrotum—the pouch in the male which contains the testes.

Semen—the fluid secreted from the testicles and accessory male organs, e.g. prostate.

Semivegetarian—a person who eats fruits, vegetables, dairy products, eggs, and a small selection of poultry, fish, and other seafood. These individuals do not consume any beef of pork.

Sexually transmitted infection—is an infection (bacterial, parasitic or viral) that is transmitted during vaginal, oral anal sexual activity or in some cases by simply touching an infected area.

Sickle-cell anemia—an inherited chronic anemia found chiefly among African Americans, in which red blood cells become sickle-shaped due to defective hemoglobin.

Simple carbohydrates—sugars that have little nutritive value beyond their energy content.

Soluble fiber—dietary fiber which dissolves in water.

Sperm—an abbreviated form of the word spermatozoon or spermatozoa.

Spermicide—an agent that kills spermatozoa.

Sterilization—is an operation performed on the female (tubal ligation) or male (vasectomy) to permanently prevent conception.

Stress—the nonspecific response to demands placed on the body. 'Nonspecific response' alludes to the production of the same physiological reaction regardless of the type of stress placed on the body.

Stroke volume—the amount of blood pumped with each heartbeat.

Stroke—the vessels that supply the brain with nutrients become damaged or occluded and the brain tissue dies.

Symphysis—joint of the pubic bones in the female.

Syphilis—a serious bacterial infection caused by the spirochete Treponema pallidum. This sexually transmitted infection can have three stages and be fatal.

Systemic circulation—the part of the circulatory system that moves blood between the heart and the rest of the body.

Tar—by product of burning tobacco; dark sticky substance which contains carcinogens.

Target heart rate zone—the range of heart rates that should be reached and maintained during cardiovascular endurance exercise to obtain training effects.

Testes—the reproductive glands inside the scrotum which are also referred to as testicles. Sperm and hormone production are the two main functions of the testes.

THC—Tetrahydrocannabinol; active ingredient in marijuana.

Thrombosis—the intravascular formation of a blood clot.

Tolerance—a condition in which an individual adapts to the amount of alcohol consumed to experience the same effects.

Triglyceride—an ester derived from glycerol, the chief component of fats and oils.

Tuberculosis—an infectious disease characterized by the formation of tubercles in body tissue; primarily affecting the lungs.

Ulcer—an open sore on the skin or some mucous membrane, discharging pus.

Unsaturated fats—fats derived primarily from plant products.

Urethra—the passage from the bladder through which urine is excreted.

Uterus—the hollow, pear-shaped muscular organ into which the ovum is received through the fallopian tubes and where it is retained during development and from which the fetus is expelled through the vagina. When a female is not pregnant it is about the size of a fist.

Vagina—a sheath; the canal from the cervix to the vulva.

Vas deferens—a long tube through which sperm travel during ejaculation.

Vegans—true vegetarians. Their diets contain absolutely no meat, chicken, fish, eggs, or milk products.

Venae cavae—the large veins through which blood is returned to the right atrium of the heart.

Ventricles—the two lower chambers of the heart from which blood blows through arteries to the lungs and other parts of the body.

Virus—any of a large group of tine infective agents causing various diseases.

Vitamins—organic substances that are necessary for normal body metabolism, growth, and development.

Vulva—the external female genitalia.

Water-soluble vitamins—vitamins not stored in the body for a significant amount of time. Amounts that are consumed and not used relatively quickly by the body are excreted through urine and sweat. Examples include the B vitamins and vitamin C.

Wellness—a process of making informed choices that will lead one, over a period of time, to a healthy lifestyle that should result in a sense of well-being.

Index